The Brain Aneurysm

Vini G. Khurana & Robert F. Spetzler

Bloomington, IN

authorHOUSE®
Milton Keynes, UK

AuthorHouse™
1663 Liberty Drive, Suite 200
Bloomington, IN 47403
www.authorhouse.com
Phone: 1-800-839-8640

AuthorHouse™ UK Ltd.
500 Avebury Boulevard
Central Milton Keynes, MK9 2BE
www.authorhouse.co.uk
Phone: 08001974150

First published by AuthorHouse 11/20/2006

ISBN: 978-1-4259-5708-7 (e)
ISBN: 978-1-4259-5707-0 (sc)

Library of Congress Control Number: 2006907567

Printed in the United States of America
Bloomington, Indiana

This book is printed on acid-free paper.

The Brain Aneurysm

A comprehensive resource for brain aneurysm patients, their families, and physicians

Vini G. Khurana, MBBS, BSc(Med), PhD

Robert F. Spetzler, MD, FACS

Division of Neurological Surgery
Barrow Neurological Institute
St. Joseph's Hospital and Medical Center
Phoenix, Arizona

Correspondence: Robert F. Spetzler, MD
Barrow Neurological Institute
350 W. Thomas Road; Phoenix, AZ 85013
Ph: 602 406 6037; Fax: 602 406 4195
E-mail: barbara.hecht@bnaneuro.net

Acknowledgments

The authors thank Nancy Spetzler for reading the original manuscript, Mr. Mark Schornak, MS, for providing illustrations, and Shelley Kick, PhD, for editorial assistance. The authors are grateful to Mr. Michael Hickman, Mr. Craig Carnell, and Ms. Marie Clarkson for their assistance with the animations and operative imaging. The authors also thank Ms. Judy Wilson, Ms. Jaime Hoffman, and Ms. Barb Hecht for their help in the production and submission of this work, and gratefully acknowledge the staff of St. Joseph's Hospital and Medical Center, Catholic Healthcare West, and the Barrow Neurological Institute, Phoenix, Arizona.

Dedication

This book is dedicated to the countless lives affected and taken by brain aneurysms. Half of the proceeds from this book will be donated to cerebrovascular research.

Disclaimer

While it is the intention of the authors that this book represents a comprehensive, accurate and useful resource for people interested in brain aneurysms, it should be noted that the material it contains does not necessarily reflect the opinions, practices, or protocols of any given organization, institution, department, or individual. This text should be used as a useful adjunct to other available medical and educational resources related to brain aneurysms. It should not be used as an alternative to personal consultation with a physician.

Abbreviations

AVM	Arteriovenous malformation
CBF	Cerebral blood flow
CSF	Cerebrospinal fluid
CT	Computerized tomography
CTA	Computerized tomographic angiography
DVT	Deep venous thrombosis
eNOS	Endothelial isoform of nitric oxide synthase
ICP	Intracranial pressure
ICU	Intensive care unit
MRA	Magnetic resonance angiography
MRI	Magnetic resonance imaging
NO	Nitric oxide
SAH	Subarachnoid hemorrhage
TBI	Traumatic brain injury
TIA	Transient ischemic attack
URL	Universal resource locator

Table of Contents

CHAPTER 1.
Why does one need to know about all of this, anyway?

Brain aneurysms occur in as many as one in 20 people in most societies and thus represent a global problem. Most of these aneurysms will never be detected and will never cause a problem. However, every year, 30,000 people in the United States alone and hundreds of thousands worldwide suffer the dreaded complication of a brain aneurysm, namely, rupture. This condition is also known as aneurysmal SAH.

A ruptured brain aneurysm is an unforgiving entity. Unlike most medical conditions, a brain aneurysm ruptures suddenly, usually without warning, and takes away or severely disables precious lives swiftly and without remorse. The human and economic costs of this disorder are staggering. Although physicians have long known about aneurysms and although technologies for their detection and treatment have improved, the overall outcome of aneurysmal SAH remains dismal. More than half of the people who seek treatment for a ruptured aneurysm will survive less than 6 months. Many of the survivors will not return to independent living. For these reasons, it is important to increase awareness about these brain lesions and the symptoms that they cause, about when individuals should be evaluated, about how aneurysms are treated, and about what to expect after diagnosis and treatment of an aneurysm. The goal of this book is to increase such awareness.

For individuals diagnosed with an unruptured brain aneurysm and for those who survive their rupture, knowledge about these entities is a precious commodity. Insight about brain aneurysms and their complications can empower patients and their family members by helping them to make informed decisions during their treatment and recovery.

CHAPTER 2.
About brain arteries

To understand what a brain aneurysm is, readers must first understand brain arteries and how they function. Therefore, this chapter describes the structure, organization, and function of brain arteries.

The structure of brain arteries

Brain arteries can be likened to steel cylindrical pipes, each consisting of a wall enclosing a hollow space known as the lumen. Blood, which is composed of liquid serum and blood cells, normally flows in the lumen under pressure derived from the pumping action of the heart and the stiffness of the arterial wall. If the wall of a blood vessel ruptures, say from a ruptured brain aneurysm or other vascular malformation, blood can spurt from the lumen. Some large brain arteries course through a space on the surface of the brain known as the subarachnoid space.

The wall of a brain artery has three major layers and six main components (**Figure 1**). The three main layers of an artery are the intima, the thin innermost layer closest to the lumen; the media, the relatively thick middle layer of the wall; and the adventitia, the outermost layer. Between the intima and the media is a thin layer of elastic tissue known as the elastic lamina. Arteries elsewhere in the body have two layers of elastic tissue, an inner layer between the intima and media, and an outer layer between the media and adventitia. The elastic lamina has many naturally occurring openings, which are called perforations.

The six main components of a blood vessel wall are endothelial cells, collagen fibers, elastic fibers, smooth muscle cells, fibroblasts, and nerve fibers. The smallest of brain vessels, known as brain capillaries, have two other cell types: astrocytes and pericytes. Astrocytes are supporting cells in the brain that send their foot processes out and over the capillary wall. Pericytes are cells scattered along the capillary wall whose function is unknown. The intima of brain arteries is composed of a single layer of cells known as the endothelium. This layer rests on a protein-rich layer called the basal lamina. Moving outward across a blood vessel wall, one

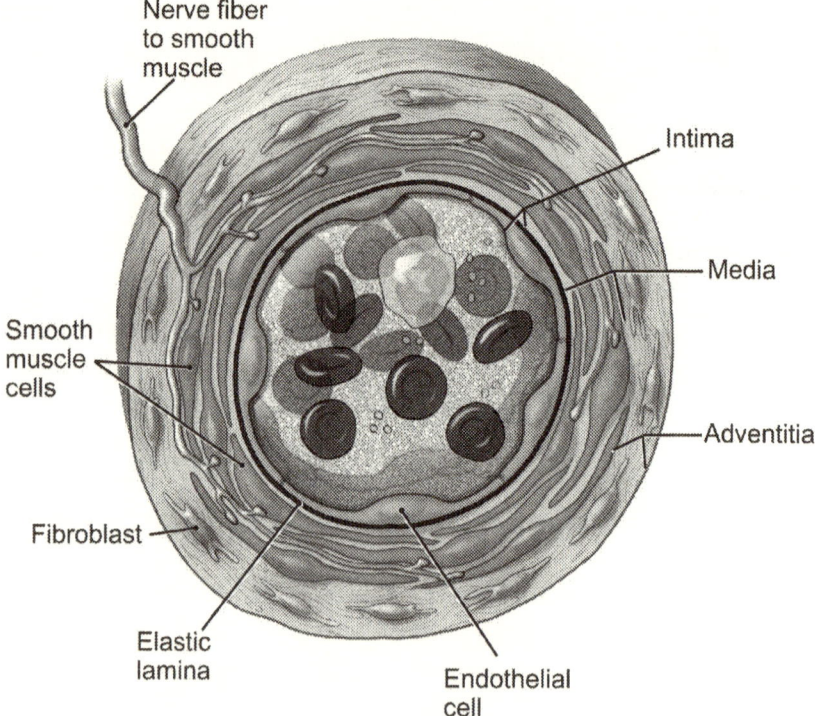

Figure 1. Structure of a normal brain artery. A section across the wall of a brain artery, which has been cut like a loaf of bread, shows the layers and cells that compose the wall of a blood vessel. *With permission from Barrow Neurological Institute.*

would first encounter the elastic lamina rich in elastin protein. Next, the media composed of smooth muscle cells would be encountered. The last layer encountered would be the adventitia, composed of both fibroblasts, which produce fibrous collagen protein, and nerve fibers, which supply the smooth muscle cells.

The organization of brain arteries

Four main arteries or trunks enter the brain from the neck. The two internal carotid arteries enter at the front under the surface of the brain, and the two vertebral arteries enter at the back under surface of the brain. From the ends of these trunks arise a ring of arteries that encircles the undersurface of the brain. This ring is known as the circle of Willis (**Figure 2**). In as many as 40 to 45% of people, this "ring" is

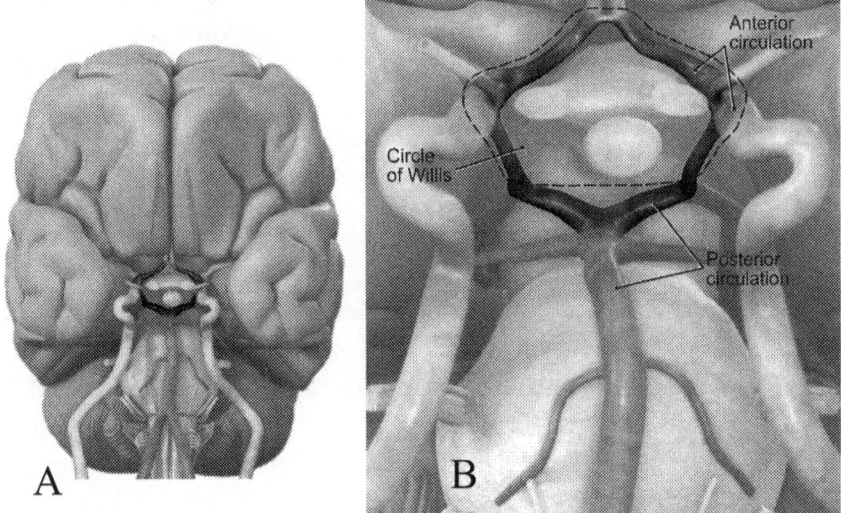

Figure 2. The circle of Willis. (A) Overview of the undersurface of the brain shows the major arteries in this region. (B) Together, these arteries form the circle of Willis. The arteries in the top part of the figure (*inside broken line*) are collectively referred to as the anterior circulation. The arteries in the bottom part of the figure (*below broken line*) are collectively referred to as the posterior circulation. All of these arteries lie in the subarachnoid space. *With permission from Barrow Neurological Institute.*

not a complete circle, but this finding is regarded as a normal variation of brain vessel anatomy.

Branching from or part of the circle of Willis are vessels known as the anterior cerebral arteries, anterior communicating artery, middle cerebral arteries, posterior communicating arteries, carotid termini, posterior cerebral arteries, and apex of the basilar artery. From these vessels, tiny critical arterial branches known as perforators arise. These perforating arteries supply vital deep structures of the brain and brainstem. Also arising from the larger arteries at the base of the brain are small arteries known as pial arteries. Pial arteries course over the surface of the brain (known as the cortex) and dip into the brain's valleys (sulci), which lie between its cliff edges or gyri. From the pial arteries many smaller arterioles exit, usually at right angles to their parent vessels, and perforate into the deeper substance of the brain. The arterioles end in capillaries, which drain first into venules, and then into larger veins. The veins drain into very high-volume, low-pressure venous systems known as dural venous sinuses. These high throughput venous channels eventually empty into the internal jugular veins in the neck, which empty into the right atrium of the heart.

How brain arteries function

The job of a brain artery is to allow nutrients in the blood to reach and perfuse the target tissue, the brain. In fact, at any given time, a fifth of the heart's output is directed toward the brain. Veins complete this circuit by draining metabolic waste products from the brain. The job of carrying blood from the heart to and through the brain is not a simple or passive process. That is, blood vessels are not merely a set of rigid, inert tubes connecting two organs. Blood flow to the brain, also referred to as CBF, is a complex and active process subject to stringent control. The normal regulation of CBF is an integrated process that involves all layers of the walls of blood vessels and the compartments in the brain filled with fluid. An adequate description of how CBF is regulated therefore must include endothelial, myogenic, neurogenic, neuroglial, and metabolic mechanisms. This technical process is addressed in **Chapter 24**.

CHAPTER 3.

What is an aneurysm?

When a region of a wall of a blood vessel weakens, it can balloon outward to form a sac-like structure. This structure is called an aneurysm, a word derived from the Greek, *aneurysma*, meaning a widening (**Figure 3**).

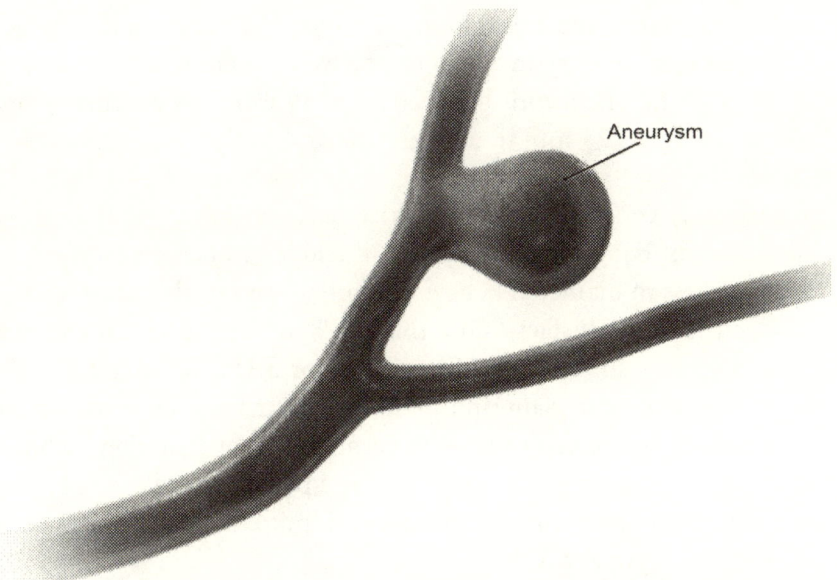

Aneurysm

Figure 3. A brain aneurysm. A brain artery with an outpouching. This outpouching, which may be referred to as a sac, blister, or small balloon, is an aneurysm. *With permission from Barrow Neurological Institute.*

A saccular or berry aneurysm is the most common type of aneurysm. It is the aneurysm typically referred to in discussions of brain aneurysms. These berry aneurysms look like sacs or berries sticking from the side of a blood vessel wall. Most berry aneurysms have a neck region. As described in **Chapter 5**, berry aneurysms tend to grow and rupture. Most of this book is concerned with saccular aneurysms, the problems that they cause, their treatment, and recovery from aneurysmal SAH.

The fusiform aneurysm is less common than the berry aneurysm. Unlike the saccular aneurysm, a fusiform aneurysm looks like a blood vessel that is expanded or ectatic in all directions. A fusiform aneurysm is typically associated with fatty plaque or atherosclerosis in the artery, or with an injury or break in the arterial wall. Fusiform aneurysms do not have a neck region, and they seldom rupture (**Chapter 21**).

Aneurysms can also be classified according to their size. Small aneurysms, those with a diameter of 10 mm or less, are the most common. The diameter of giant aneurysms is 25 mm or more. In between, that is, from 11 to 15 mm and from 20 to 24 mm in diameter are the "large" and near-giant" aneurysm sizes, respectively. There is a gray area of classification for aneurysms between 16 to 19 mm. Of all aneurysms, 95% are less than 25 mm in diameter. That is, only 5% are "giant."

Interestingly, certain differences exist between aneurysms of these different sizes. For most purposes, small and large aneurysms, together 15 mm or less in diameter, behave in similar ways in that they tend to grow and rupture. In fact, more than 90% of aneurysms in this size range become symptomatic with rupture or SAH. In contrast, 75% of patients with near-giant and giant aneurysms are admitted to the hospital with symptoms caused by compression or irritation of brain structures surrounding the aneurysm. The remaining 25% of patients with near-giant and giant aneurysms are admitted to the hospital after suffering aneurysmal SAH.

Most brain aneurysms arise from the parent arteries, or their main branches, forming the circle of Willis (**Chapter 2**), and most tend to occur in the anterior (front) brain circulation. It is well known that most aneurysms form near regions where an artery branches. At these regions, referred to as bifurcations, the turbulent forces exerted on the arterial wall by the flowing blood may be the greatest. These branch points are also where fatty plaques most tend to be deposited. It has also been suggested that brain blood vessels naturally may be slightly weaker at such points.

CHAPTER 4.
Vital statistics

How common are brain aneurysms?

As many as 5 to 10% of the general population may have one or more brain aneurysms. Others have suggested that this number may be less than half of 1%. In the United States, with a population of about 300 million people, these percentages mean that 1.5 million to 30 million people may harbor an aneurysm. Most reports suggest that the prevalence of brain aneurysms is between 1 to 5%.

Not all aneurysms cause problems. On average, there are 10 cases of aneurysmal rupture per 100,000 people per year. That is, aneurysmal SAH has an incidence of 10 per 100,000 per year. This statistic has often been misquoted. It does not mean that 10 of 100,000 aneurysms rupture. Rather, it means that every year, for every 100,000 people in the community-at-large, 10 people can be expected to be hospitalized for a newly diagnosed ruptured brain aneurysm. Therefore, in the United States, about 30,000 people are diagnosed with a ruptured brain aneurysm per year. Although ruptured aneurysms are relatively uncommon, they represent a very serious illness. Aneurysmal SAH is associated with a high rate of death (mortality) and disability (morbidity).

Table 1. Main Risk Factors for Aneurysm Formation

Smoking

Hypertension

Previous Aneurysm

Family History of Brain Aneurysm

Connective Tissue Disorder

Older than 40 Years

Female

Blood Vessel Injury or Dissection

The natural history of a condition refers to the typical chain of events that can be expected in the course of an illness if no treatment is given. The natural history of aneurysmal SAH is often devastating. In the absence of treatment, half to two-thirds of all patients who suffer a brain hemorrhage from a ruptured aneurysm will die within 6 months. Half of the remaining survivors are unable to return to work or to maintain an independent life. With heightened community awareness, earlier diagnosis through better imaging, the future prospect of genetic testing for brain aneurysm rupture risk (**Chapter 24**), and more and improved treatment options (**Chapter 10**), the chances of patients with brain aneurysms of attaining a good outcome are higher than ever before.

What are the risk factors that lead to aneurysm formation?

Several risk factors increase the likelihood of an aneurysm forming (**Table 1**). Smoking is an extremely important risk factor for aneurysm formation. A history of high blood pressure or hypertension, a previous aneurysm in the same person, or a positive family history, where one or more close (first-degree) relatives such as a parent or sibling was diagnosed with a brain aneurysm, are also important risk factors. In fact, 5 to 15% of people diagnosed with a brain aneurysm also have a relative with a brain aneurysm. Age and gender are also risk factors. People older than 40 years tend to be diagnosed with brain aneurysms more often than younger people. Most of these patients are women. Occasionally, children also have brain aneurysms. Several reports have cited a higher incidence of brain aneurysm rupture among Japanese than among other ethnic groups. Otherwise, no solid scientific trends indicate that one ethnic group or race is more likely to develop an aneurysm than any other group.

A person suffering from or having a first-degree relative with an inherited connective tissue disorder, such as polycystic kidney disease, alpha-1 anti-trypsin deficiency, Marfan's syndrome, Ehlers-Danlos syndrome, or neurofibromatosis Type 1, has a high risk of forming a brain aneurysm. People born with abnormal blood vessel connections in the brain, referred to as congenitally abnormal cerebrovascular anatomy, and those with a history of brain vessel injury from head trauma may also have an increased risk of aneurysm formation later in life. Inflammation of blood vessel walls, referred to as vasculitis, is an another risk factor.

Each risk factor contributes to the weakening of a region of the wall of a brain artery. This weakening, in turn, permits an aneurysm to form.

Pregnancy and aneurysm formation and rupture

Pregnancy has not been established as a risk factor for the formation or rupture of an aneurysm. Of course, a brain aneurysm in women can rupture any time, including during pregnancy. Wherever possible, aneurysm surgery should be avoided during the first trimester of pregnancy. There is no substantial evidence to support that a residual or incompletely treated, unruptured aneurysm will grow or rupture during pregnancy, although in theory either of these events can occur.

Are brain aneurysms inherited?

About 10% of brain aneurysms appear to run in families; the rest are considered sporadic. That is, most brain aneurysms appear to occur spontaneously. However, new genetic evidence (**Chapter 24**) suggests that some genetic factor may predispose even sporadic aneurysms to rupture. These new data do not necessarily imply that there is an inherited tendency for brain aneurysms to rupture. Rather, they imply that the tendency for an aneurysm to rupture may be influenced by parts of an individual's genetic code.

CHAPTER 5.

Development of brain aneurysms

Like most diseases, aneurysms (**Figure 4**) may be congenital or acquired. If congenital, an affected individual may have been born with a defect in the wall of an artery in the brain, with an abnormal communication in the brain circulation, or with a hereditary disease that led to and worsened a defect in an arterial wall. If acquired, some event or illness during the affected individual's life led to the development of the aneurysm. The congenital theory once was thought to be the most important factor, and it still may be in people with inherited connective tissue diseases that weaken arterial walls. However, most brain aneurysms are now thought to be acquired. Perhaps the most significant reasons are smoking, which is associated with injury to the endothelium of blood vessels (**Chapter 2**), and high blood pressure, which stresses the walls of the blood vessels. In individuals with a strong family history of brain aneurysms, some yet unidentified, inherited genetic defect might predispose them to form brain aneurysms. This genetic predisposition may be compounded by the added insults of smoking and hypertension.

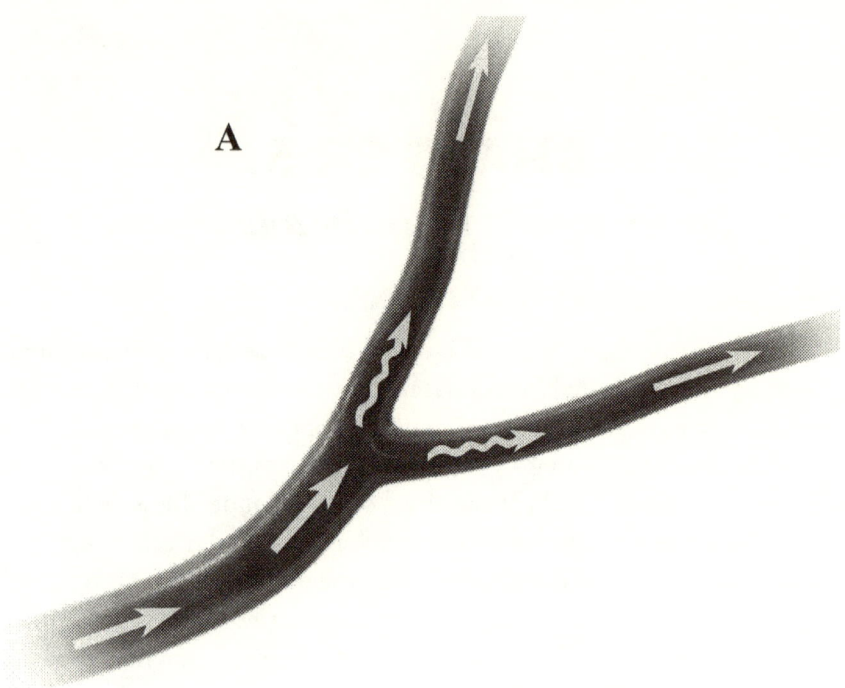

Figure 4. Brain aneurysm development. (A) A normal arterial branch point with normal blood flow (*straight arrows*) in the artery. No aneurysm is present, but normal turbulent flow (*wavy arrows*) occurs at and beyond the branch points. *With permission from Barrow Neurological Institute.*

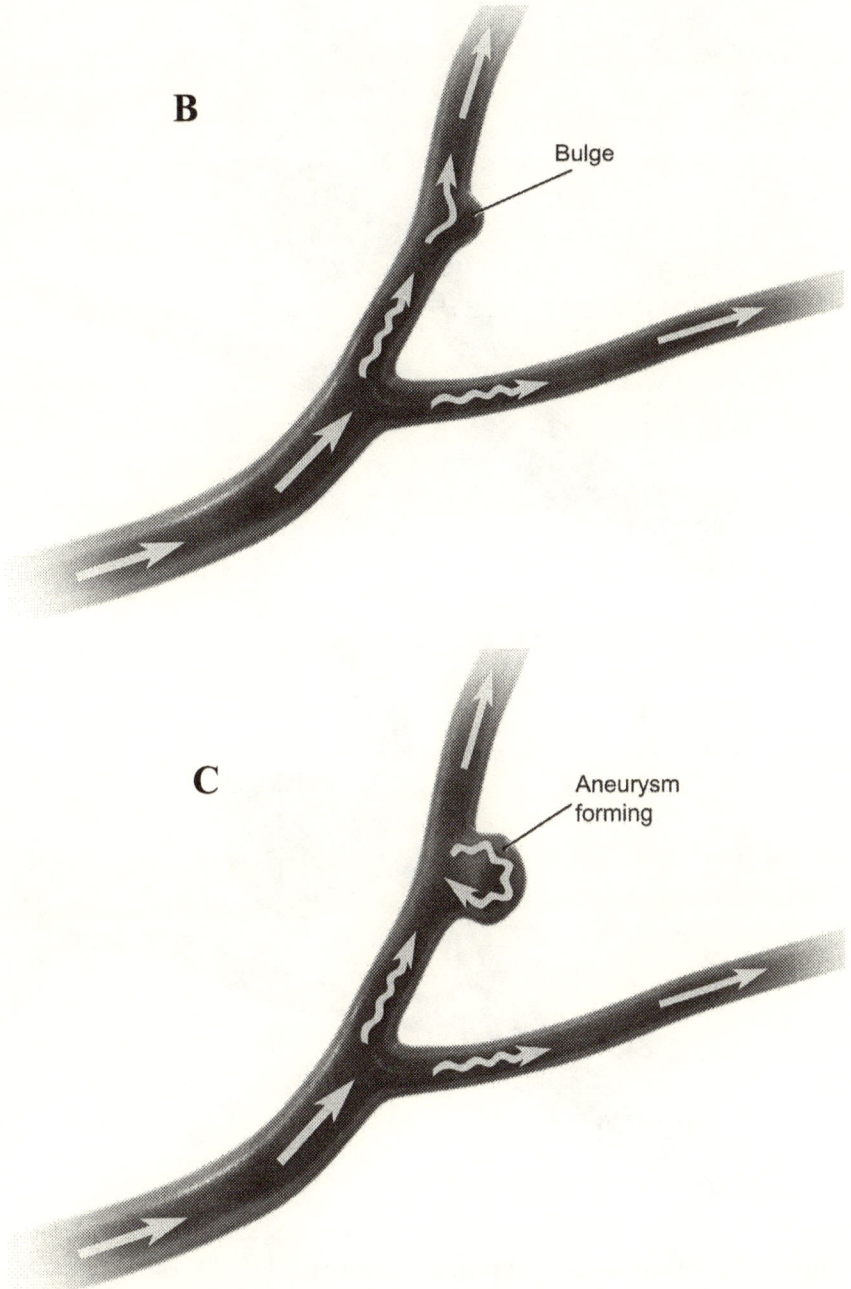

Figure 4. Brain aneurysm development. (B) An aneurysm starts to develop on one side of the arterial wall and (C) expands over time. *With permission from Barrow Neurological Institute.*

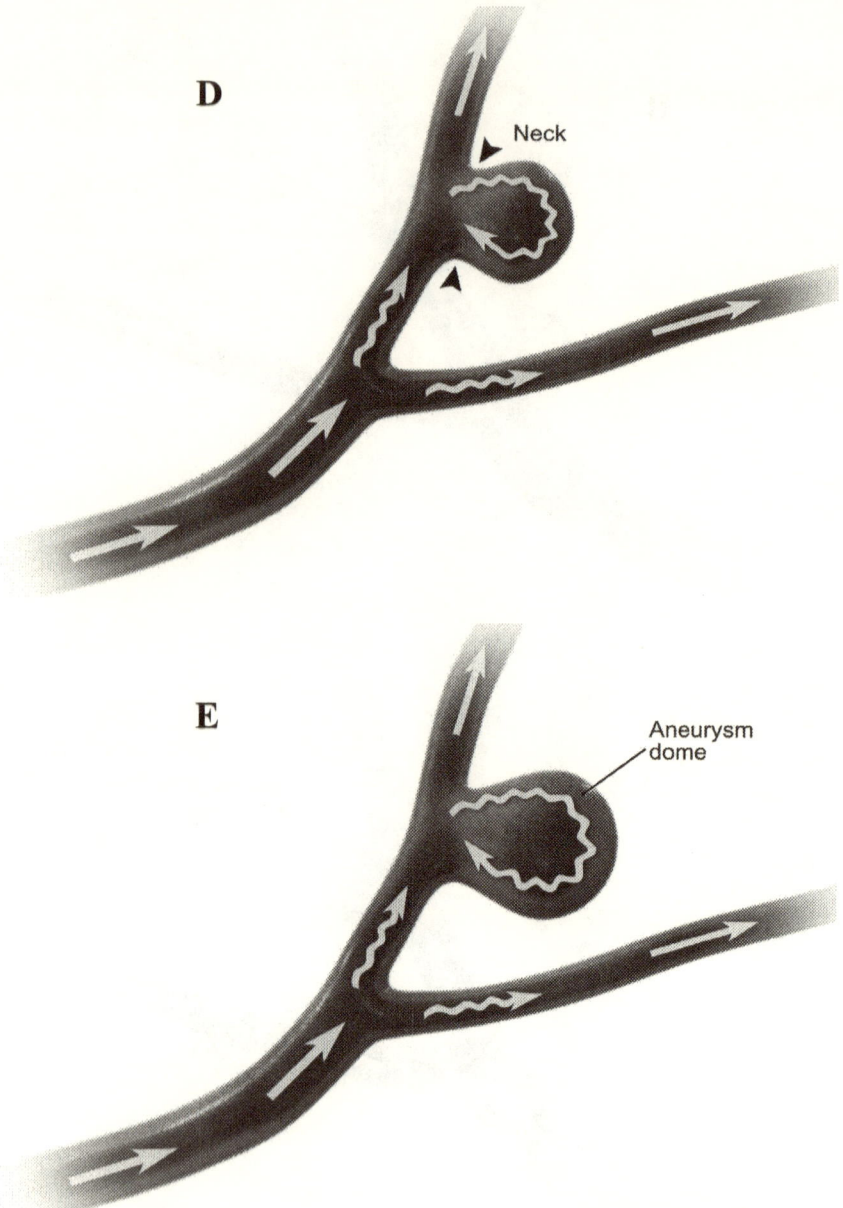

Figure 4. Brain aneurysm development. (D) As the aneurysm enlarges, a "neck" may become apparent (*arrowheads*). Blood flow in the body or sac of the aneurysm (*curved wavy arrow*) becomes more and more turbulent. (E) The turbulence leads to progressive weakening of the aneurysm wall, especially at the top or dome of the aneurysm. *With permission from Barrow Neurological Institute.*

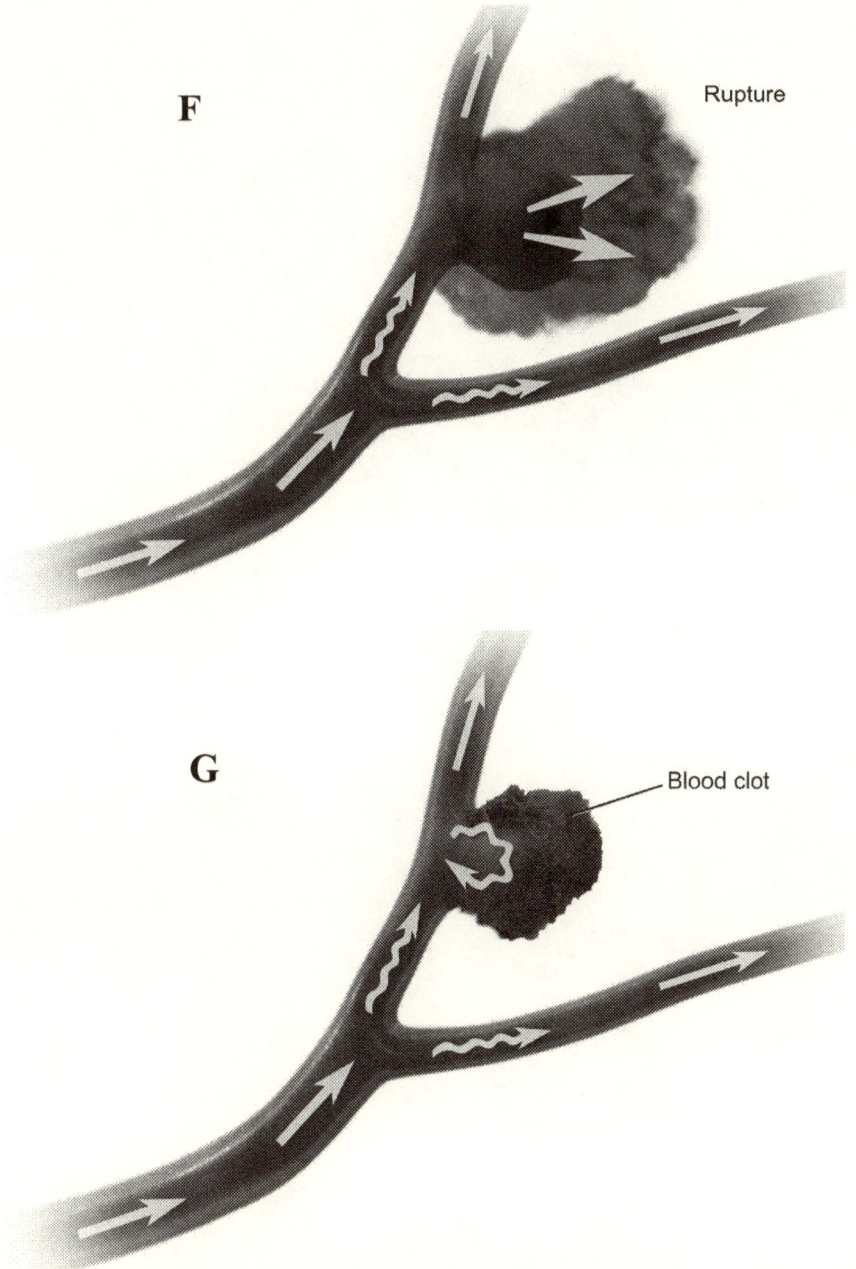

Figure 4. Brain aneurysm development. (F) Eventually, the aneurysm ruptures. (G) Blood gushes from the artery and enters the subarachnoid space where it forms a clot. This event is referred to as SAH. *With permission from Barrow Neurological Institute.*

CHAPTER 6.
Symptoms

Most aneurysms are silent. The person is totally unaware of a problem until the aneurysm ruptures. This is the pattern of events in about 90% of all aneurysm patients. At the time of rupture, the person experiences one or more of the following symptoms: a sudden, extremely severe headache, which may be described as the "worst headache" of one's entire life or as a "sledge-hammer" headache that struck like a "bolt of lightening;" vomiting; neck stiffness; collapse or loss of consciousness; sudden loss of function in one or more parts of the body like a classic stroke; or a seizure.

In 3% of patients, the aneurysm may be found by chance, that is, incidentally. In 7% of patients the aneurysm is found because of symptoms caused when its relatively large size (mass) compresses or irritates surrounding brain structures. Patients with "mass effect" may have symptoms such as continuous morning headaches, nausea, vomiting, or excessive drowsiness. Loss of function in one or more of one of the nerve bundles in the brain or brainstem can lead to symptoms such as weakness of facial muscles, double vision, impaired balance or hearing, tongue deviation, or weakness in the limbs. Seizures and stroke-like events have also been reported. All of these symptoms can also be associated with conditions unrelated to aneurysms such as brain tumors. Any individual with such symptoms—regardless of age—should undergo immediate and careful evaluation by a physician.

Warning leak

Some aneurysms do not frankly rupture; instead, they may tear a little and release a small amount of blood. Such small warning leaks occur in 15 to 30% of patients before their aneurysm actually ruptures. A warning leak often causes sudden and severe headache that may be associated with some degree of neck stiffness. The warning leak can occur anytime before the actual "main bleed."

Brain attack

The American Heart Association and its Stroke Council coined the term "brain attack" (**Chapter 23**) to describe the brain equivalent of the common "heart attack." The term encompasses the symptoms of a stroke, many of which were mentioned above. The stroke itself may arise from blockage of a blood vessel, which is the usual cause, or from the rupture of an aneurysm. The concept is important, aimed at increasing community awareness about this important and potentially life-threatening brain condition.

CHAPTER 7.
Complications

Once an aneurysm ruptures, time becomes of the essence. About 10% of people with ruptured aneurysms die instantaneously from the volume or mass effect of the hemorrhage in the brain or from cardiac arrest, in this case, known as "cardiac stunning." In the surviving 90% who reach an emergency room alive, the most feared complication, especially hours to a few days after the initial event, is another hemorrhage. Other complications of the aneurysmal rupture include a heart attack or arrhythmia, cerebral vasospasm, hydrocephalus, and seizures. Any new neurological impairment, such as muscle weakness or paralysis, or speech or language dysfunction, is referred to as a neurological deficit. Ruptured aneurysms frequently cause such deficits.

Rebleeding

Consider the example of a patient with an unruptured aneurysm. As of yet, the aneurysm has an intact wall and has never leaked, bled, or hemorrhaged. One day, however, the weakened aneurysm wall, usually the dome region, suddenly gives way. This event is referred to as a bleed, hemorrhage, or SAH. After the rupture, the aneurysm wall is surrounded by blood clot. The clot can stop the bleeding, but it is relatively fragile. It can rupture again, causing a second SAH. This event is referred to as aneurysmal rebleeding, or rehemorrhage. A single aneurysm can hemorrhage multiple times.

Although not all aneurysms rupture and not all ruptured aneurysms rerupture, aneurysmal rupture and rerupture are still relatively frequent and potentially life-threatening events. If a patient survives the initial hemorrhage, the chances of surviving a rebleed are even less. Therefore, the major problem associated with rebleeding is the lowered likelihood of survival.

Why do aneurysms rebleed? Basically, aneurysms rebleed because their thin, ballooned-out walls, which were weak to begin with (**Chapter 2**), are much weaker after the initial rupture (**Figure 5**). The wall of a recently ruptured aneurysm continues to experience stress from the normal pounding of blood still flowing through the parent artery from which the aneurysm arose. That hammer-like stress, which amounts to increased pressure on the aneurysm wall, predisposes the aneurysm to rebleeding. Therefore, in patients with hypertension affecting the brain's arteries, the risk of rebleeding can be expected to be high.

If the flow of blood slows in the aneurysm lumen, a clot or "thrombus" may form. This event, referred to as thrombosis, can happen before or after the initial rupture. The clot, which is often a hard and craggy mass, may exert additional stress on the wall of the aneurysm and make it easier for the wall to be torn or retorn, particularly if the normal pulsations of blood are transmitted through the mass itself. Before or after rupture or rerupture of an aneurysm, small channels of blood can form in the thrombus, a phenomenon referred to as recanalization. Recanalization is also associated with growth, rupture, and rerupture of an aneurysm. Finally, the cells that make up the wall of an aneurysm depend on oxygen and other nutrients for their survival. If their nourishment is cut off by the growth or rupture of an aneurysm, the wall is further weakened as its cells effectively starve and die.

There are three important facts about the risk of rebleeding. First, all ruptured aneurysms, regardless of their original size, are at risk of rebleeding. Second, the presence of blood clot in a ruptured giant or near-giant aneurysm does not protect the patient from another hemorrhage. Third, the risk of rebleeding gradually increases with time from the initial rupture. Therefore, as a rule of thumb, the earlier an aneurysm is treated the better it is for the patient.

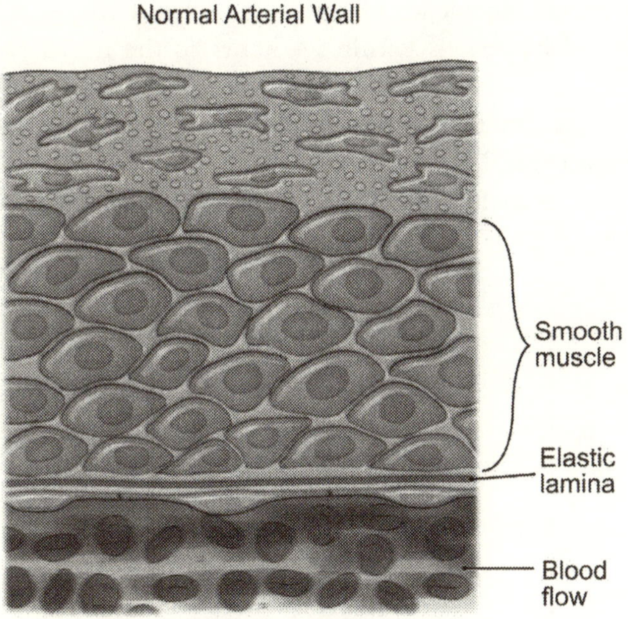

Normal Arterial Wall

Smooth
muscle

Elastic
lamina

Blood
flow

Aneurysm Wall

Smooth
muscle

Elastic
lamina

Blood
flow

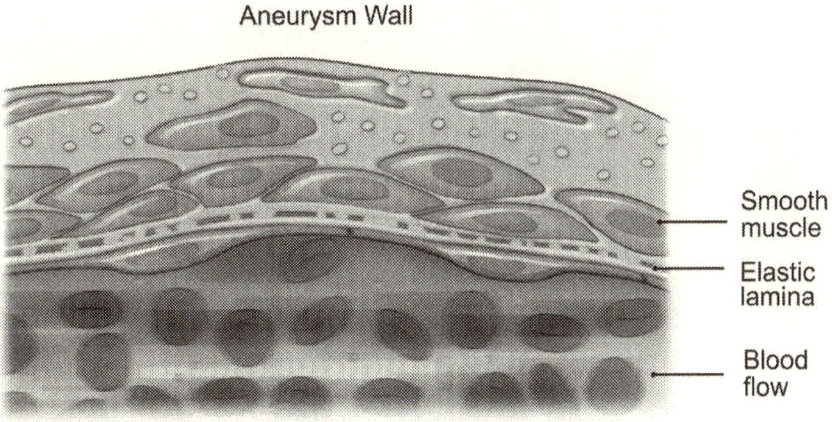

Figure 5. Why aneurysms rebleed. (A) The layers of a normal arterial wall in the brain compared with a (B) much thinner and weaker aneurysm wall before its initial rupture. Both walls are drawn to the same scale. The wall of the aneurysm has only sparse elastic tissue and a thin layer of muscle. The aneurysm wall is likely to be even more fragile after SAH. *With permission from Barrow Neurological Institute.*

When is an aneurysm most likely to rebleed? Most studies suggest that the highest incidence of rebleeding from a ruptured aneurysm, regardless of its size, is within 24 hours of the initial hemorrhage. During this period, 4% to 10% of patients with a ruptured aneurysm will experience another hemorrhage. The daily rate of rebleeding then decreases to 1% to 2% for the first 2 weeks. Therefore, a patient's overall chance of experiencing another hemorrhage within 2 weeks of the initial hemorrhage is 20% to 25% (**Figure 6**).

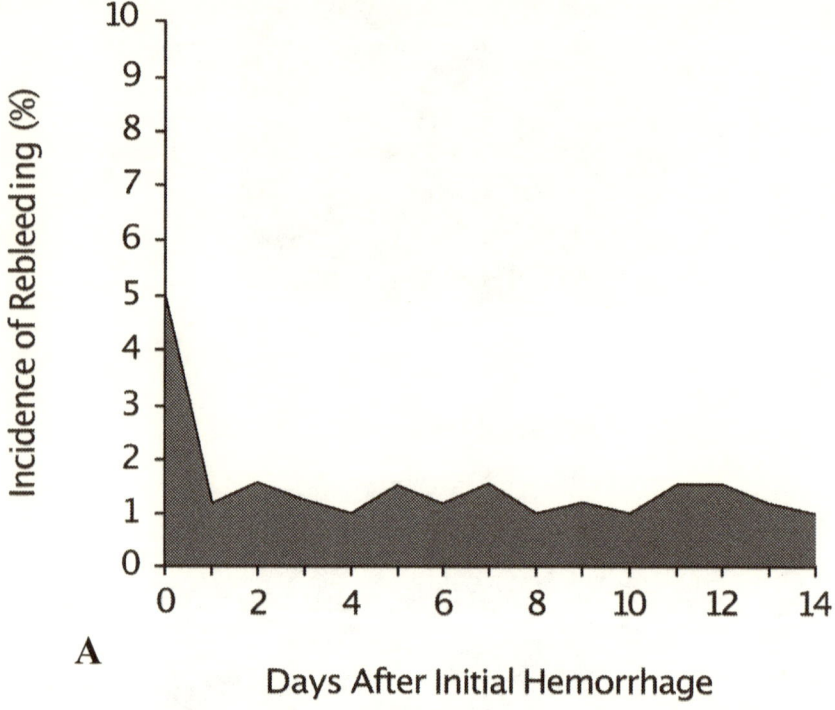

Figure 6. Pattern of aneurysmal rebleeding. (A) The incidence of aneurysmal rebleeding from the day of the initial hemorrhage (Day 0) to 2 weeks after this event, and (B) the cumulative rate of rebleeding during the first 2 weeks after the first hemorrhage. Incidence refers to the percentage of patients experiencing a rebleed event on any given day after the initial bleed (Day 0). Cumulative rate refers to the overall percentage of patients experiencing a rebleed by a given day after the initial bleed (Day 0). *With permission from Barrow Neurological Institute.*

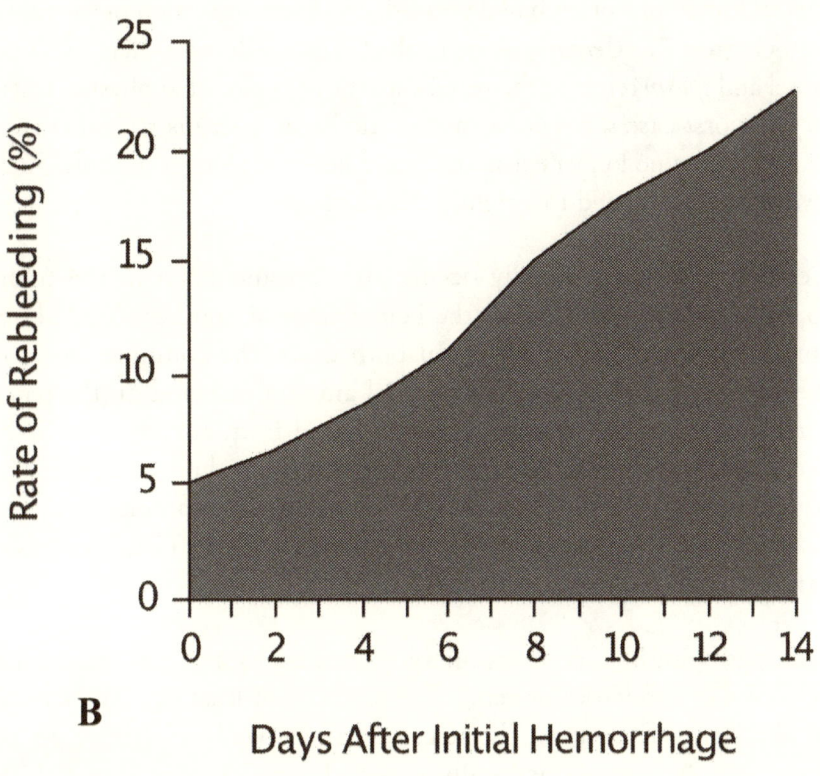

B

Days After Initial Hemorrhage

What are the complications of rebleeding? The feared consequences of aneurysmal rebleeding are death and serious disability. Clinical reports indicate that 4 of 10 patients who suffer a rebleed from a previously ruptured brain aneurysm will not survive the rebleed event. Most of those who do survive a subsequent hemorrhage are left with serious neurological impairments, and many are unable to return to independent living. Given that even a first aneurysmal bleed carries a high risk of death and permanent disability, the overall chance of a given patient surviving two bleeds from the same aneurysm is low. Early diagnosis and, where appropriate, early referral to an experienced neurosurgical center for thorough planning and early treatment are key recommendations for patients with ruptured brain aneurysms.

Cerebral vasospasm

Cerebral vasospasm is a term that refers to physical narrowing of the central lumen of a brain blood vessel due to overcontraction of the vessel wall (**Figure 7**). *Cerebral* refers to the brain, while *vaso* refers to blood vessel and *spasm* refers to the vessel's spastic or constricted physical state. In the worst-case scenario, a vasospastic brain artery is so constricted that its lumen no longer exists and blood flow is no longer possible. Such a state can be likened to a tightly clenched fist.

Cerebral vasospasm usually occurs after an aneurysm in the brain ruptures or, very rarely, after the hemorrhage of another blood vessel abnormality such as an AVM. In both cases, the common factor is the abnormal presence of a substantial amount of blood on the outer surface of the blood vessel. In theory, blood from any cause of SAH can trigger vasospasm. Cerebral vasospasm is also known to occur in patients who suffer SAH from TBI sustained, for example, in motor vehicle or sporting accidents. In patients with severe TBI, vasospasm can negatively influence outcomes.

Vasospasm is thought to occur only in arteries and not in smaller arterioles or capillaries or veins. The reason is at least partially related to physical differences in the structure of the walls of these types of vessels. Arteries have thick walls, especially because they have a thick smooth muscle layer, and can clamp down or contract harder than veins or capillaries. Molecular differences among these vessels also may partly explain why vasospasm occurs selectively in arteries. Vasospasm occurs in the large arteries composing the circle of Willis and the main branches arising from this vascular ring. It even occurs in the small pial arteries that course over the surface of the brain.

Vasospasm can be classified into three types: subangiographic, angiographic, and clinical vasospasm:

Subangiographic vasospasm cannot be detected by cerebral angiography, the best imaging method for detecting vasospasm. In other words, vasospasm is occurring at a physical level, but it cannot be detected radiologically because of limitations of the available imaging methods.

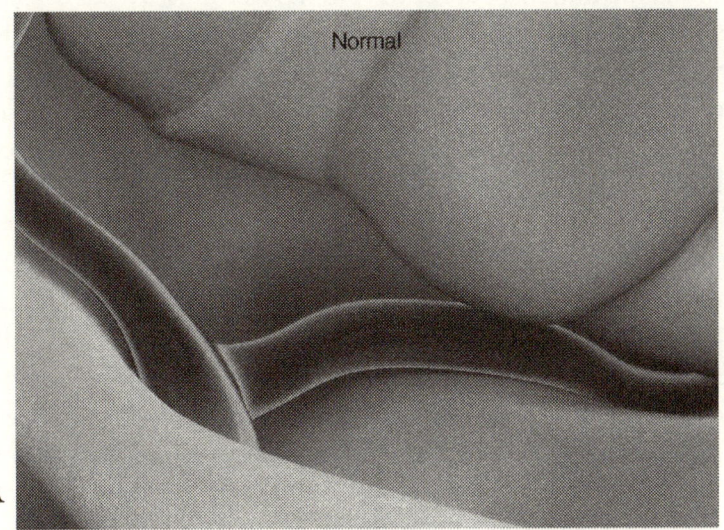

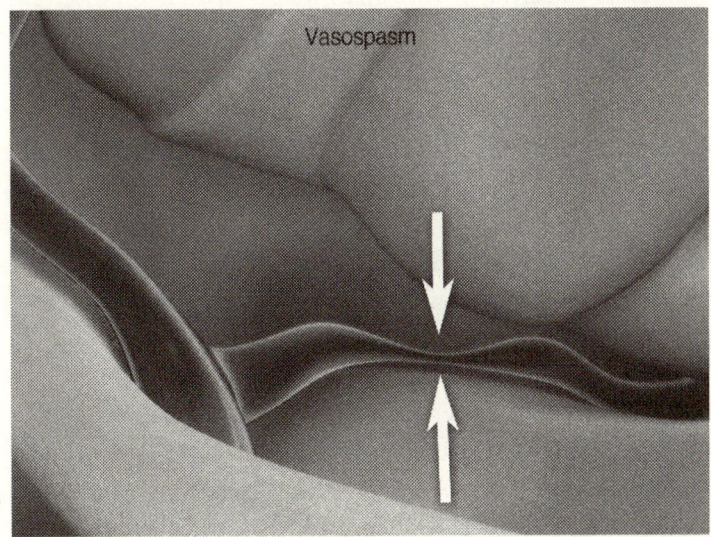

Figure 7. Vasospasm. (A) An artery with a normal diameter. (B) In vasospasm, the same artery overcontracts and becomes spastic. The central lumen of the artery, which normally permits the free flow of blood, becomes very narrow (*arrows*) and may even close entirely. This can result in a stroke. *With permission from Barrow Neurological Institute.*

Specifically, either the arterial narrowing is too mild to detect, or the spasm is happening in a part of the arterial tree that is most difficult to image with angiography—the smaller brain arteries. A patient may or may not be clinically affected by subangiographic vasospasm. That is, at the bedside, a physician may or may not be able to detect its presence. Some patients with subangiographic spasm, however, do have detectable symptoms.

Angiographic vasospasm can be detected by cerebral angiography. It is thought that if vasospasm can be detected angiographically, then the patient should have related symptoms that a physician can detect at the patient's bedside. However, not all patients with angiographic vasospasm experience symptoms from its occurrence. The reasons are unknown but may relate to the genetically determined capacity of the brain of different individuals to tolerate the same degree of arterial spasm. Alternatively, this observation may be explained by differences among patients in terms of the "road-map" of their brain circulation. For example, some patients may have back-up routes of blood supply, which is referred to as their collateral circulation. When detected, vasospastic arteries caused by aneurysmal bleeding tend to be close to the site of the ruptured aneurysm. However, more distant arteries can also be vasospastic in a "diffuse" or "generalized" manner.

Clinical vasospasm, regardless of a patient's angiographic findings, can be detected by a physician conducting a physical examination of a patient.

Most, if not all, patients suffering aneurysmal SAH will experience some degree of subangiographic vasospasm triggered by the presence of blood in the subarachnoid space. Angiographic vasospasm tends to be most readily detected by cerebral angiography about 7 days after the SAH. However, it may be detected as early as 3 days after the hemorrhage. Depending on when angiography is performed, angiographic vasospasm occurs in half to two-thirds of all aneurysm patients. Clinical vasospasm occurs in about a third of all patients with aneurysmal SAH. Typically, the arterial narrowing associated with cerebral vasospasm is a temporary event that lasts a few days to 3 weeks. Even though vasospasm is reversible, it can still be harmful, or even fatal.

Is there a genetic predisposition for developing vasospasm? It has long been known that the amount of blood seen on a CT scan after the rupture of a brain aneurysm correlates with the risk of developing cerebral vasospasm. That is, the more blood that it is present, the higher is the patient's risk of developing cerebral vasospasm. It has also been observed that different patients with similar amounts of blood on a CT scan may or may not share the same susceptibility to vasospasm or its effects. For example, Patient A and Patient B both have ruptured brain aneurysms. They also have the same amount of blood on their CT scans based on a physician's evaluation. However, Patient A develops cerebral vasospasm while patient B does not. Alternatively, Patient A develops only angiographic vasospasm while patient B develops both angiographic and clinical vasospasm. In the absence of significant differences between age, race, gender, medical illnesses and so forth, how can this paradox be explained?

Differences in certain vasoregulatory or vasoresponsive genes and proteins between Patient A and Patient B may underlie the difference in their response to vasospasm. One such candidate is the key vasoregulatory molecule, referred to as eNOS. Such differences between patients are called genetic polymorphisms. Polymorphisms are not mutations; rather, they are relatively common genetic variations that occur across populations. Researchers from Japan first identified a link between polymorphic eNOS and susceptibility to coronary or heart vessel vasospasm. This particular polymorphism is called the T-786C eNOS promoter single nucleotide polymorphism. This polymorphism also predicts susceptibility to cerebral vasospasm after rupture of a brain aneurysm (**Chapter 24**). More studies are needed before T-786C eNOS becomes a benchmark for clinical or genetic screening.

What is the mechanism of cerebral vasospasm at a molecular level? The precise mechanism underlying cerebral vasospasm is unknown. What is known, however, is that the cascade of events leading to abnormal constriction of the artery (**Figure 8**) begins with oxyhemoglobin, a breakdown product of red blood cells. Oxyhemoglobin is derived from the blood clot that forms in the subarachnoid space after an aneurysm ruptures. Oxyhemoglobin leads to the generation of so-called reactive oxygen species, which are related to oxygen-derived free-radicals such

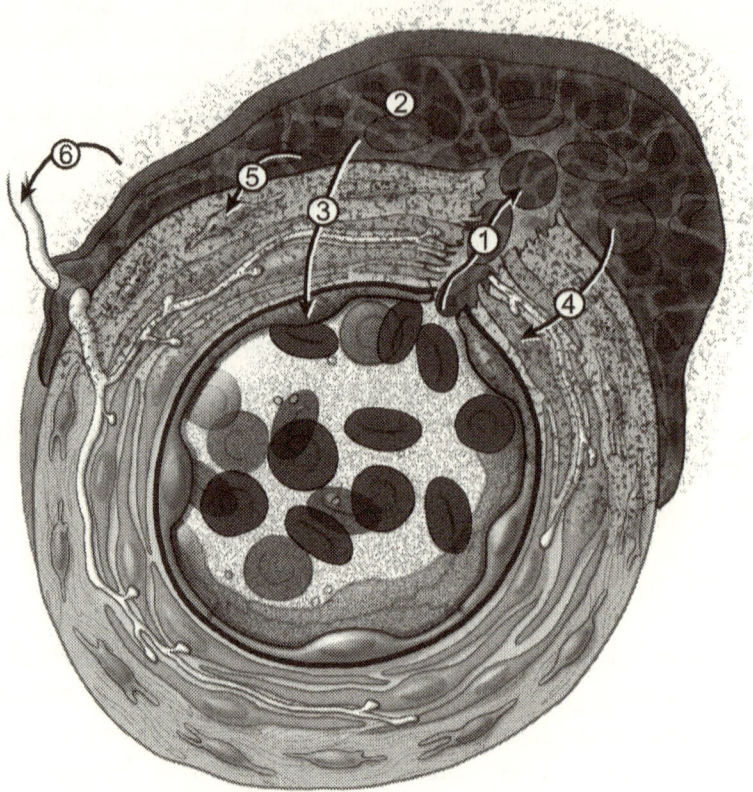

Figure 8. Mechanism of cerebral vasospasm. A section of arterial wall is shown, similar to the cross-section shown in **Figure 1**. This part of the wall represents the wall of a brain aneurysm that has just ruptured. Blood gushes from its normal compartment in the lumen of the blood vessel through the (1) ruptured wall and into the subarachnoid space. There, it forms a (2) clot, which contains many red blood cells and, eventually, their breakdown products, especially oxyhemoglobin. These products generate free radicals, which damage cells in all layers of the blood vessel wall, including the (3) endothelium, (4) smooth muscle, and adventitia. In the adventitia, (5) fibroblasts and (6) nerve fibers are damaged. A brisk inflammatory reaction follows. Overall, the blood vessel overcontracts, its lumen shuts down, and local cerebral blood flow is impaired. *With permission from Barrow Neurological Institute.*

as superoxide ($O_2.$). These species are toxic and damage cells in the wall of neighboring blood vessels, including endothelial cells, smooth muscle cells, and adventitial fibroblasts. They also damage nerve fibers. The damage disturbs the artery's vasomotor function, that is, its normal cycle of relaxation and contraction. The artery reacts by shutting down or contracting in an abnormal manner. This process partially explains how cerebral vasospasm occurs. In theory, as SAH becomes worse, more oxyhemoglobin is generated. The blood vessel wall then becomes more damaged and the severity of cerebral vasospasm worsens (**Chapter 24**).

Why is cerebral vasospasm a problem? The function of arteries in the brain is to transport blood and all its nutrients to a specific part of the brain. Vasospasm causes an artery to lose the ability to perform this crucial function. As a result, the part of the brain normally supplied by the vasospastic artery effectively starves, a process referred to as ischemia. If the ischemic region of the brain is starved long enough, it may die, an event known as infarction or stroke. So even though cerebral vasospasm is a transient phenomenon, it can still damage the brain irreversibly or cause death. Overall, cerebral vasospasm accounts for about 20% of the severe disability and death associated with ruptured aneurysms. Even though aneurysmal rebleeding is the most dreaded complication in patients surviving a ruptured aneurysm, the next most feared complication is vasospasm.

What are the symptoms (what a patient describes) and signs (what a physician observes on physical examination) of cerebral vasospasm (**Table 2**)? The least threatening symptoms are fever, a stiff neck, and mild confusion. More severe symptoms include dysphasia, an impaired ability to comprehend language and to communicate, including speech, and hemiplegia, a profound weakness down one side of the body. As vasospasm worsens, a patient's consciousness may become severely impaired. Ultimately, the most severe event is the classic picture of a stroke, which can involve one or more of the features discussed above. These symptoms and signs can wax and wane, that is, come and go with different degrees of severity for days. Their onset is usually at least 3 days after the bleed. They last as long as 3 weeks.

Table 2. Clinical Picture of Cerebral Vasospasm

Fever

Neck Stiffness

Mild Confusion

Dysphasia

Hemiplegia

Severely Impaired Consciousness

Classic Picture of "Stroke"

How is cerebral vasospasm detected? Vasospasm can be detected by physical examination of the patient and by imaging methods such as cerebral angiography and transcranial Doppler ultrasonography. During cerebral angiography, an opaque dye is injected into the blood stream of a patient. The dye is usually injected through a catheter or thin piece of tubing inserted into the femoral artery in the groin. The dye eventually reaches the blood vessels in the brain. At this point, radiographs are taken. The dye is radio-opaque, that is, x-rays do not pass through it as easily as they do through neighboring brain tissue. Therefore, the dye stands out. This test provides a roadmap of the brain circulation, which shows a physician the course of arteries, their pattern of communication, their length and diameter, and the presence of any abnormalities. On a cerebral angiogram, vasospastic arteries appear to have abnormally thin columns of blood in their lumens, almost string-like in their width.

A brain CT scan in a patient suspected of having vasospasm may show new strokes in the distribution of the vasospastic artery or arteries. An MRI study of the brain may localize the extent of the brain tissue damaged by vasospasm even more precisely. MRA can show vasospasm in large vessels, but at present cerebral angiography is the most reliable tool for this purpose.

Transcranial Doppler ultrasonography is a bedside test that relies on ultrasound waves generated from a probe placed on the scalp to detect the flow of blood in a cerebral artery. It is convenient, noninvasive, safe, and effective and can be used to rapidly confirm clinical findings. However, ultrasonography has numerous technical limitations and the information it provides is seldom of the same caliber as that obtained from angiography. Nonetheless, physicians now use this test regularly to follow patients with a ruptured aneurysm for the development and progression of vasospasm.

How is vasospasm treated? Over the last 40 years, various silver bullets have been proposed to be the cure for cerebral vasospasm. Unfortunately, the cure still remains elusive, most likely because the precise cause of cerebral vasospasm at a molecular level is unknown. At present, there are two important aspects to the medical management of a patient at risk of, or suffering from, vasospasm. First, such patients need to begin taking a drug called nimodipine early. Second, where possible, the principles of hypervolemic hypertensive hemodilution therapy must be followed.

Nimodipine is a calcium-channel blocker. It dilates or relaxes arteries by blocking the entry of calcium ions into vascular smooth muscle cells. It also may be neuroprotective, that is, it may directly protect brain neurons from injury. Nimodipine is administered orally, several times daily, for about 3 weeks after a hemorrhage occurs.

Hypervolemic hypertensive hemodilution therapy means that the fluid levels and therefore blood pressure or, more correctly, the mean arterial pressure, of a vasospasm patient are kept relatively high and the concentration or viscosity of the patient's blood is kept relatively low. Together, this pattern of blood properties improves CBF. This form of therapy, however, is associated with its own risks, particularly if a patient's aneurysm has not been clipped surgically or treated by endovascular coiling. In such cases, hypervolemic hypertensive hemodilution therapy can increase the risk of aneurysmal rebleeding.

Other methods used to dilate or relax a vasospastic artery on an emergency basis involve the use of a catheter. For example, a strong vasodilating agent such as papaverine can be delivered directly into the territory of the vasospastic artery to dilate the artery. Alternatively, a catheter can be used to wedge a balloon into the vasospastic artery. The balloon is then inflated but not released from the tip of the catheter. Doing so dilates the artery mechanically. This technique is referred to as mechanical angioplasty. Papaverine therapy often works, but its effects are short-lived. Mechanical angioplasty can also be effective. However, the artery can rupture during angioplasty, and normal arterial function is never restored. Catheter-based techniques are reserved for severe vasospastic emergencies.

The most helpful treatment to prevent vasospasm is to clip an aneurysm as soon as possible and to remove as much of the subarachnoid blood products as possible. However, excessive manipulation of blood vessels during surgery can increase their risk of going into spasm. Aggressive CSF blood clearance using an external ventricular drain, a lumbar drain, or both are also helpful in treating patients with significant SAH.

On an experimental front, gene therapy is being explored as a potential treatment option for cerebral vasospasm (**Chapter 24**). A genetically engineered vector carrying the gene for eNOS is delivered to a vasospastic territory. The intention is to dilate the artery by causing the local overproduction of NO, a potent dilator of blood vessels. Another method is to infuse a NO-containing solution directly into the brain circulation either through the traditional catheter-based endovascular approach or by direct delivery into the CSF via a spinal tap. These experimental procedures are still being evaluated but appear promising.

Once the precise cause of vasospasm is understood, it is likely that the most appropriate therapy will then be developed. In the meantime, careful monitoring, nimodipine, and hypervolemic hypertensive hemodilution therapy are the best that can be done for patients.

Hydrocephalus

The brain contains spaces called ventricles, which are filled with CSF. This fluid, produced by structures collectively referred to as the choroid plexus, circulates throughout the brain. CSF exits the brain near the brainstem and courses over the surface of the brain in the subarachnoid space or into and around the spinal cord. In the lowest part of the spine, just above the level of the tailbone, is a generous CSF-filled cavity known as the lumbar cistern. During a spinal tap or lumbar puncture, CSF is drawn from this cistern. CSF is mostly absorbed at the top surface of the brain in structures called arachnoid granulations (**Figure 9**).

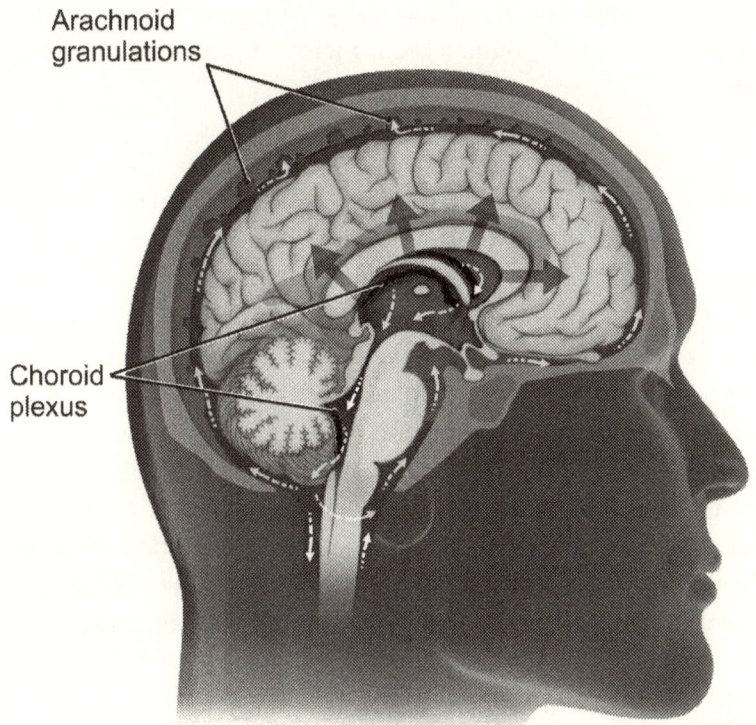

Arachnoid
granulations

Choroid
plexus

Figure 9. Development of hydrocephalus. The CSF-filled spaces in the brain are known as ventricles. CSF circulates through and around the brain (*white dashed arrows*) and is absorbed over the top of the brain through the arachnoid granulations. Disrupting the absorption of CSF by blood products at the arachnoid granulations, for example, by aneurysmal SAH, can lead to symptomatic hydrocephalus as the accumulating CSF exerts pressure on the surrounding brain tissue (*large dark arrows*). *With permission from Barrow Neurological Institute.*

When a brain aneurysm ruptures, the blood, which should be on the inside of blood vessels, now occupies the subarachnoid space and eventually reaches the arachnoid granulations. Cells and debris in the blood can clog up and damage these relatively delicate structures, obstructing the absorption of CSF. This damage can be short term or permanent. The accumulating CSF enlarges the ventricles through backpressure, just like a dam effect. This condition is referred to as hydrocephalus or water on the brain. As pressure builds in the brain, it causes one or more of the following symptoms: headache, nausea, vomiting, blurred or double vision, increasing drowsiness, coma, and death.

Hydrocephalus is treated by diverting the CSF. First, CSF is temporarily diverted through a special drainage tube. When placed in the ventricles, the tube is called an external ventricular drain. When placed in the lumbar cistern, the tube is called a lumbar drain. CSF intermittently drains through this tubing. After several days, an attempt is made to gradually clamp off or "wean" the drain to determine if the natural pathways for CSF absorption have recovered. If so, the drain is removed. If a drain cannot be weaned successfully, that is, the patient becomes symptomatic from hydrocephalus each time the drain is clamped, a shunt usually needs to be placed by the neurosurgeon. A shunt, which serves as a permanent drain, requires a separate operation. One in three patients with a ruptured brain aneurysm develops hydrocephalus, and many of these patients will require placement of a permanent shunt.

Seizures

Seizures are the brain's equivalent of heart arrhythmias. That is, seizures represent disordered communication or circuitry among neurons. Seizures related to the presence or rupture of a brain aneurysm are common, probably occurring in about 10% of all patients with a brain aneurysm. Irritation or disruption of brain tissue by blood from aneurysmal SAH can cause seizures. In theory, a large or growing unruptured aneurysm can also cause seizures by direct irritation of brain tissue. Less frequently, seizures appear after surgery for brain aneurysms. Such seizures may be related to direct pressure placed on the brain by retraction as the surgeon attempts to eradicate the aneurysm.

Seizures are treated with anti-seizure medications such as phenytoin, carbamazepine, and barbiturates. All anti-seizure medications have side effects, which can include one or more of the following: skin rash, dizziness or wooziness, imbalance, nausea, vomiting, drowsiness, and a risk to the fetus in pregnant patients. When seizures do occur in aneurysm patients, they usually subside quickly and the length of treatment is usually short (i.e., days to a few months). An aneurysm patient rarely requires long-term anti-seizure medication. The use and blood level of these medications should be monitored periodically by the patient's neurologist or prescribing physician.

Cardiac stunning

The rupture of a brain aneurysm can affect the heart, although the patient may not feel this effect. Sometimes, the disturbance is mild as seen on an electrocardiogram or heart rhythm strip in the emergency room or ICU. However, at other times, the heart disturbance is not only symptomatic but potentially life-threatening. About 5% of newly admitted patients with a ruptured brain aneurysm develop a significant new heart problem at the time that a brain aneurysm ruptures. In fact, among individuals with ruptured brain aneurysms who die from aneurysmal SAH before reaching medical attention, a significant number may be caused by a life-threatening arrhythmia or a frank heart attack at the time of rupture. Exactly how the heart problem occurs is unknown. The presence of sudden, excruciating head pain may be a contributing factor, but the occurrence of a massive discharge from the autonomic or sympathetic nervous system at the time of rupture or rerupture has also been implicated. The presence of chest tightness, pressure, or a new pain involving the chest-jaw-arm axis should be promptly communicated to a physician. Conversely, a physician should always consider this scenario when assessing patients with aneurysmal SAH.

Sodium and fluid imbalance

There is a known association between the rupture of an aneurysm and the impairment of sodium levels and fluid balance. Such patients often have two patterns of sodium and fluid imbalance. The first pattern is referred to as cerebral salt wasting. Cerebral salt wasting is thought to be related to the leakage of salt and water from the body due to the increased presence or activity of naturally occurring diuretic hormones in the body called natriuretic peptides. Somehow, aneurysmal SAH triggers these small protein components to increase the loss of sodium and fluid via the kidneys into the urine. Patients with cerebral salt wasting thus become depleted of fluid and sodium.

The second pattern of imbalance is referred to as the syndrome of inappropriate antidiuretic hormone secretion. In this condition, a naturally occurring hormone called antidiuretic hormone or vasopressin is oversecreted, overactive, or both. Antidiuretic hormone is derived from the part of the brain known as the hypothalamus and is secreted from its adjoining pituitary gland. Oversecretion of antidiuretic hormone causes the kidneys to resorb more water. As a result, the sodium in the blood becomes diluted and its level drops.

The precise trigger for either cerebral salt wasting or syndrome of inappropriate antidiuretic hormone secretion pattern is unknown. Cerebral salt wasting is more common in patients with a ruptured aneurysm than syndrome of inappropriate antidiuretic hormone secretion. Regardless of their causes, physicians caring for such patients must carefully monitor their sodium levels and fluid balance. A drop in sodium can cause confusion, delirium, seizures, coma, or death. The treatment is beyond the scope of this book.

CHAPTER 8.
Detection

Sadly, most aneurysms are detected only after they have ruptured. Recall that in fewer than 10% of patients, an aneurysm is detected by chance or, in the case of bigger aneurysms, due to symptoms arising from compression of nearby brain structures.

Cerebral angiography is frequently used to detect brain aneurysms. If there is no clot in an aneurysm, it lights up on an angiogram like a sac coming off the parent artery. Sometimes the lumen of the aneurysm is filled with clot, a common finding in large aneurysms. In such cases, angiography may not show the real extent of the aneurysm.

Other advanced radiographic imaging methods for detecting aneurysms are MRI and its associated method, MRA. These methods have the advantage of being less invasive than cerebral angiography—the femoral artery does not need to be punctured, and tubing does not need to be inserted and navigated through the arterial tree. However, MRI and MRA may not detect the smallest aneurysms as well as cerebral angiography can. Furthermore, certain patients with metallic implants cannot undergo MR because of problems associated with magnetic attraction and interference referred to as ferromagnetism. Patients with implants made from nonferromagnetic hardware such as titanium or platinum can still be imaged safely and effectively by MR methods. A patient should check with his or her physician and radiologist before undergoing MRI or MRA.

Ultrasound techniques such as Duplex or Doppler ultrasonography have no role in the detection of aneurysms. However, transcranial Doppler ultrasonography can be useful for detecting vasospasm after aneurysmal SAH. Common radiography (x-ray) is not used for aneurysm detection.

A combination of CT scanning and angiography, referred to as CTA, is gaining popularity for detecting aneurysms. For this technique, an intravenous dye is injected into the patient at the time of CT scanning. Someday CTA may replace conventional cerebral angiography because the former is so much quicker, cheaper, and less invasive than the latter. The ability to create high-resolution, color, and 3-dimensional images with CTA is very helpful for surgeons planning to operate on these lesions.

After an aneurysm has been detected by one or more of the above methods, lumbar puncture is frequently used to determine whether it has already ruptured. This technique involves the insertion of a spinal needle into the lower part of the back and withdrawing some CSF. The CSF is then examined for blood pigments or xanthochromia. Xanthochromia is first present about 6 hours after SAH and may linger for weeks.

No single blood test can reliably predict the formation or rupture of a sporadic brain aneurysm. Researchers have been working on developing such a test and are waiting validation through a larger clinical trial (**Chapter 24**). Certain genetic or hereditary diseases may have genetic fingerprints that can be detected in the blood or after an appropriate tissue biopsy. When present, a specifying fingerprint may indicate that a person is at increased risk of developing a brain aneurysm.

CHAPTER 9.
Screening

Screening for brain aneurysms refers to the attempt to detect a brain aneurysm in a person who has had no symptoms related to, or previous diagnosis of, aneurysmal disease. In general, a screening method should be associated with minimal or no risks and be relatively cost-effective while providing good and accurate information. At the outset, a patient should discuss the possible benefits of screening and any risks associated with screening procedures with his or her physician or attending neurologist or neurosurgeon. At present, there are no hard and fast rules regarding screening for brain aneurysms. Some physicians consider a patient with two or more first-degree relatives known to have the diagnosis of brain aneurysm to be a strong candidate for screening. Some patients with certain inherited connective tissue diseases are also considered good candidates for brain aneurysm screening, particularly if they have had problems in other parts of their body related to their connective tissue disorder.

Screening is performed with an imaging device that scans the brain, such as an MRI scanner, particularly in its MRA mode. MRA is regarded as a safe and acceptable way of detecting brain aneurysms, although some very small aneurysms may be difficult to detect by this scanning technique. CTA is showing some promise as an alternative to MRA for brain aneurysm screening. CTA is quicker and less expensive than MRA. It also is less claustrophobic for patients than MRA. However, clinical studies are still needed to compare the effectiveness of these two methods as screening tools for unruptured brain aneurysms.

Cerebral angiography may be regarded by some physicians as an alternative method for screening. Although this procedure is the best method known for detecting brain aneurysms, it is associated with more risks than MRA or CTA. For example, on rare occasions, the catheter navigated through the body during angiography can damage distant arteries. There is also a small risk of stroke during cerebral angiography. Some patients may be allergic to the contrast material, although new contrast media have been developed to reduce this risk. Finally, cerebral angiography is relatively expensive compared with MRA and CTA.

An important question needs to be addressed when patients are screened for brain aneurysms: What will an asymptomatic patient do if a brain aneurysm is identified during screening? Will the patient be prepared to undergo the necessary investigations and possible treatment? This issue complicates the process of screening. Certainly, some aneurysms discovered by screening may have a high risk of rupturing, particularly if their diameter is 7 to 10 mm or more, or if the aneurysm is found to be growing on consecutive studies. However, small aneurysms, that is, those significantly less than 10 mm in diameter also can rupture. So, if an aneurysm that has been causing no symptoms is found incidentally by screening, should it be treated? If so, when and how? These issues require considerable discussion between the patient and the treatment team, including a neurosurgeon, neurologist, and endovascular surgeon.

CHAPTER 10.
Treatment

If an aneurysm is detected but has not ruptured, the immediate choice of treatments is controversial. Some physicians have found that an aneurysm with a diameter of 10 mm or more may have a significantly increased risk of rupturing. Others, however, have found that even smaller aneurysms, for example, 3 to 6 mm in diameter, are likely to rupture. They advocate that the 10-mm size is invalid as a basis for estimating risks and for deciding on whether to observe a patient or to pursue treatment. Observation means evaluating the patient's aneurysm periodically with repeated scans to determine if the aneurysm is enlarging. The bottom line is that each brain aneurysm should be evaluated on an individualized basis, with consideration of the patient's age; the presence of other significant medical conditions; the site, size, and shape of the aneurysm; whether the patient has a history of previous SAH; and the type of treatment proposed to be most suitable for a given aneurysm and patient.

The picture is more clear if an aneurysm has already ruptured. In this case, the options are either open surgery, which is usually recommended as early as possible after hemorrhage, or an endovascular intervention.

Surgical options

Cerebrovascular surgeons, also known as neurovascular surgeons or microneurosurgeons, perform four main types of open surgery for the treatment of aneurysms. First, a metallic clip can be placed across the neck of the aneurysm, a technique referred to as direct clipping (**Figure 10**). Clipping is the most certain method of curing an aneurysm. Second, a metallic clip can be placed across the artery feeding the aneurysm, a technique referred to as proximal or Hunterian ligation. Ligation allows an aneurysm to clot off with the hope that it will shrink or involute. Third, a metallic clip can be placed across all arteries feeding and draining the aneurysm, a technique referred to as trapping (**Figure 10**). The fourth method is surgical reconstruction of the aneurysmal portion of the artery. Reconstruction can involve cutting the aneurysm out of the affected artery and then repairing the vessel with a combination of sutures, clips, and graft material. These types of procedures are performed according to the features of an individual patient's aneurysm and vascular anatomy. For the most risky aneurysms, the surgeon may occasionally choose to perform part of the procedure while the patient's heart is stopped. The patient is placed on heart and lung bypass and cooled to relatively low temperatures, a procedure referred to as cardioplegia and profound hypothermia.

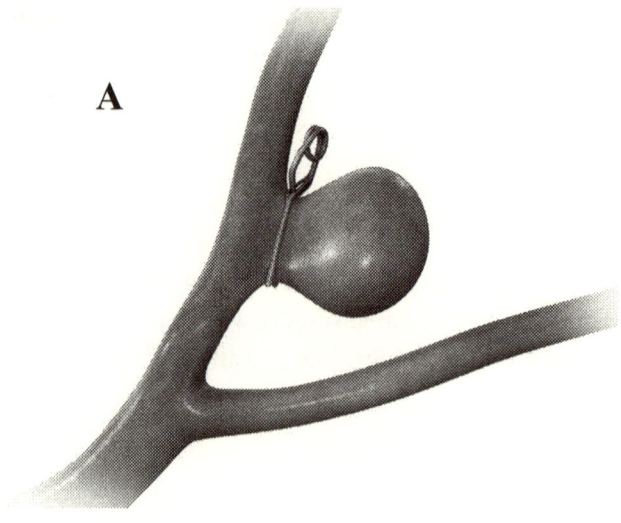

A

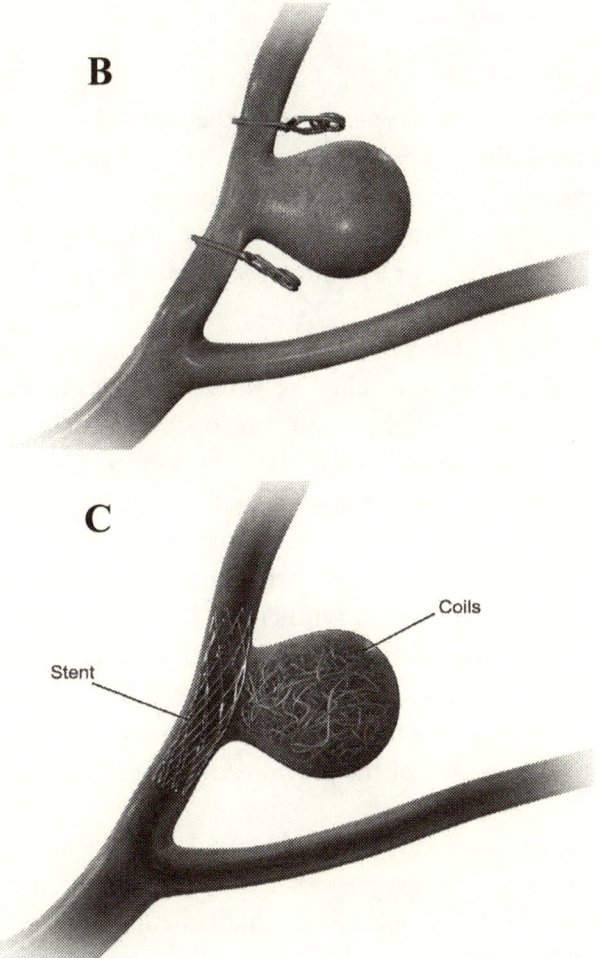

Figure 10. Techniques for treating aneurysms. (A) Direct clipping of an aneurysm. A titanium clip is placed across the aneurysmal neck, thereby effectively removing the aneurysm from the circulation. (B) Trapping of an aneurysm. Similar clips are placed on the portions of the artery that feed and drain the aneurysm. (C) A hollow stent placed by a catheter across the region of the vessel that opens into the lumen of the aneurysm isolates an aneurysm from the circulation. Through certain stents, detachable platinum microcoils can also be placed in the lumen of the aneurysm to slow down and eventually clot off its internal blood flow. *With permission from Barrow Neurological Institute.*

Endovascular options

Endovascular surgery, which does not involve open surgery, requires insertion of a catheter, typically into the femoral artery in the groin. The catheter is then navigated through the aorta and up into the brain, to the region of the aneurysm itself. The procedure is performed by a neurosurgeon who specializes in catheter techniques, known as an endovascular surgeon, or by an interventional neuroradiologist.

There are several endovascular options for treating aneurysms. First, platinum microcoils or a "glue" or similar composite material can be placed in the lumen of the aneurysm to slow the flow of blood. This option is intended to encourage the aneurysm to clot off and thereby become excluded from the parent artery. The intent is to shrink the aneurysm (**Figure 10**). Second, a balloon, with or without microcoils, can be placed in the parent artery that feeds the aneurysm, again, with the same intention. Third, a synthetic hollow bridge known as a stent can be inserted across the aneurysmal portion of the artery to cut off its blood supply. Additional coils can be placed through openings in the stent, without stopping blood flow across the open stent (**Figure 10**). Fourth, a combination of the previous three procedures can be used.

Compared to open surgery, endovascular procedures have several advantages. Open surgery is not required. The treatment can be as beneficial as surgery, especially for small aneurysms. It also can allow access to certain aneurysms that may be difficult to reach through open surgery.

In the ideal circumstance, the decision about how to best treat an aneurysm is made by joint consultation among the patient, a neurosurgeon, and an endovascular surgeon, during which the specific circumstances of the patient and aneurysm are considered carefully (**Chapter 12**). Sometimes, an aneurysm treated by coiling can persist or recur (**Chapter 19**). Subsequently, recoiling may be attempted, or open surgery may be pursued. Neither coiling nor microsurgery rule out further treatment by the same or a different means, if needed at a later time. In appropriate instances treating physicians and their patients have greatly benefited from pursuing a combined endovascular approach to brain aneurysms.

CHAPTER 11.
What a patient should think about

If an individual is fortunate enough to have been diagnosed with an aneurysm before it ruptures, many issues need to be considered, especially if treatment is recommended.

Has the patient been presented with a complete and balanced picture about treatment options?

The various treatment options and rationale are detailed in the preceding chapter.

Will the patient have the option of being treated at an experienced center by an experienced group of doctors?

Safe and effective surgery on blood vessels in the brain requires the highest level of neurosurgical training and skill and a highly sophisticated neurointensive care service. It is indisputable that brain aneurysms require expert attention and a strong commitment by physicians and patients alike during both initial care and follow-up. Reports have shown that the successful treatment of aneurysms is helped significantly by the availability of hospital resources, including appropriate intraoperative equipment, availability of an interventional or endovascular suite and neurological ICU, suitably trained nursing and paramedical personnel, and a team of appropriately trained and experienced specialists that includes microneurosurgeons, endovascular surgeons, and neurocritical care intensivists. Such resources and staff are available at most large teaching or tertiary referral centers. When possible, it behooves a patient to check with the physician regarding the microneurosurgeon or endovascular surgeon's experience in cerebrovascular surgery or endovascular therapy, respectively; the number of aneurysm patients the surgeons treats every year; and the sophistication of the hospital facility, including the mandatory presence of a neurological ICU.

To clip or coil the aneurysm?

Whether an aneurysm should be clipped or coiled is controversial, and each treatment has its proponents. The choice to clip or coil an aneurysm is based on factors specific to a given aneurysm, treating physician, available technology, patient, medical facility, and medical industry.

Aneurysm-specific factors. First, the size of an aneurysm is considered. An aneurysm 10 mm or greater in diameter is probably best treated surgically because such lesions have a relatively high rate of recurrence or persistence after an attempt at coiling. Smaller aneurysms may be amenable to either clipping or coiling. Second, the presence of multiple daughter sacs can create an awkward shape that usually warrants surgical treatment of the aneurysm. Third, the width of the neck of the aneurysm is an important consideration. The wider the neck of an aneurysm is, the more difficult it becomes to clip or coil it. Coiling through a stent may be successful, but successful surgical clipping is also frequently possible. Fourth, the location of the aneurysm is important. Aneurysms involving the posterior circulation such as the basilar artery now tend to be coiled when feasible. Fifth, if a previously coiled aneurysm has regrown, a microneurosurgeon and endovascular surgeon should be consulted to determine the best possible treatment for the regrown remnant or recurrent aneurysm. Sixth, the ease of obtaining surgical access to the neck of the aneurysm is an important aspect of the treatment decision-making process. Finally, the relationship of the aneurysm to neighboring large and small perforator blood vessels is another major consideration when deciding whether to clip or coil an aneurysm.

Physician-specific factors. Intuitively, the superspecialized training of the neurosurgeon, the surgeon's judgment, and his or her cerebrovascular experience are important in determining the outcome of aneurysm surgery. It is frequently difficult for a patient to determine this information before surgery. The Internet may be of some assistance, but the choice of surgeon often boils down to local hearsay, direct questioning, and trust. The situation is the same for the endovascular surgeon.

Technology-specific factors. Aneurysmal clipping is an enduring, time-tested, and potentially highly curative treatment. Decades of data are available on the safety and efficacy of direct clipping. Of course, open surgery is associated with risks of its own. Neither open surgery nor endovascular surgical intervention are free of risk. In the last 20 years, the evolution of the operating microscope and a large variety of aneurysm clip sizes and shapes have helped improve surgical outcomes. In comparison, endovascular treatment is still in its youth. Endovascular technology relies on coils, glues, and stents, all of which are continuing to develop rapidly. This technology is often sold as "no incision, no open operation, short hospital stay." Typically, these claims are true unless a complication arises and the assistance of a cerebrovascular surgeon is required. However, the number of neurosurgical reports of previously coiled patients who have required surgery as a salvage procedure is increasing. Many surgeons have been able to minimize head shaves, but they have not been able to eliminate the need for an incision and open operation to treat aneurysms.

Patient-specific factors. A patient may choose to have one form of treatment over another. For example, a patient may refuse any type of surgery and opt for coiling, which may indeed work out just fine. Some patients simply "want it taken care of" by open surgery, that is, without the burden of additional uncertainty and prolonged follow-up needed after coiling. Advanced age and poor medical condition may make an attempt at coiling safer than surgery by sparing the patient an operation, general anesthetic, and a longer postoperative stay in the

ICU. Sometimes, however, general anesthetics also may need to be administered for endovascular treatment.

Medical facility-specific factors. Optimally, all brain aneurysms would be treated at centers of cerebrovascular excellence. In reality, however, the outcome of a patient with an unruptured or ruptured aneurysm may partially reflect the hospital at which the patient is first treated, and the choice is usually based on geographic proximity alone. As elaborated earlier, the availability of a 24-hour on-call, highly specialized medical team is the hallmark needed to provide such patients their best chance of attaining a good outcome. Such teams are usually present at large teaching hospitals. Typically, these centers can offer both endovascular and open surgical options. Complex aneurysms needing a consensus regarding best possible treatment should be discussed among several colleagues in a multidisciplinary manner.

Media-specific factors. Media hype is an unexpected factor that can influence treatment considerations. Members of the media may perceive a new technology as a breakthrough without a deeper understanding of how the technology may translate to patient care, and of how individualized and comprehensive the analysis of brain aneurysm patients should be. Unless opinions are sought from a multitude of experienced proponents of both clipping and coiling, such reports may be biased.

Medical industry-specific factors. Developing new technologies that may affect hundreds of thousands of people worldwide every year can be lucrative. Large companies may spend considerable time and money on research and development of technology. Understandably, these companies want their investment to pay off. That is not to say that the technology may not work or be suitable. Although a given technology may be excellent for many patients, it is unlikely to be suitable for all aneurysm patients. When physicians recommend treatment, patients should be aware of conflicts of interest or any hidden agenda of big business or self-interest groups.

Postrupture considerations

A patient whose aneurysm has ruptured is unlikely to have the luxury of time to research treatment options. After an aneurysm ruptures, it needs to be treated in a timely manner to prevent fatal rebleeding (Chapter 7). The method of treatment depends on factors mentioned elsewhere (Chapter 10). Complications of aneurysmal SAH become a major consideration (Chapter 7). If the patient is comatose, both physicians and families have many other issues to address (Chapter 17).

CHAPTER 12.

What a treating physician should think about

As William J. Mayo, one of the founders of the Mayo Clinic stated: "The best interest of the patient is the only interest to be considered." When it comes to a patient with one or more unruptured brain aneurysms, the following issues must be considered carefully.

Is the aneurysm symptomatic? That is, is it causing the patient any neurological problems or complaints? Headaches, seizures, cranial nerve palsies or dysfunction, limb weakness, and hydrocephalus have all been described in brain aneurysm patients. After a careful history, physical examination, and appropriate imaging (**Chapter 8**) of the patient are obtained, the physician should be able to determine if the aneurysm is symptomatic. If it is, treatment is favored.

Treatment should also be considered for an asymptomatic aneurysm that has a diameter of 10 mm or more, or that has an irregular shape (**Chapters 10** and **Chapter 11**).

If the patient has a history of rupture from a previous separate aneurysm, a family history of aneurysmal SAH, or an inherited connective tissue disorder associated with a predisposition toward growth of brain aneurysms, treatment of a newly diagnosed aneurysm may be favored, even if the lesion is small.

Should an aneurysm be clipped or coiled? This choice remains a complex decision (**Chapter 11**). The factors favoring both treatments should be weighed carefully by the referring doctor and discussed by the treating physicians. There are no long-term data on the outcome of aneurysm coiling versus open surgery. However, clinical trials, for example, the International Subarachnoid Aneurysm Trial (**Chapter 24;** URL: http://www.surgery.ox.ac.uk/nvru/isat), are ongoing.

International Subarachnoid Aneurysm Trial is a multicenter, randomized trial comparing clipping and coiling in patients with ruptured brain aneurysms. Originally, almost 10,000 aneurysmal SAH patients were eligible for inclusion in this study. However, 78% of these patients were excluded either because they refused to participate (9%) or because their aneurysms were considered not to be equally amenable to treatment by either technique (69%). Because almost all brain aneurysms can be clipped surgically, some authors have argued that the exclusion of such a large proportion of patients from the International Subarachnoid Aneurysm Trial indicates that coiling is less suitable than open surgery for the treatment of most brain aneurysms.

In brief, the International Subarachnoid Aneurysm Trial found that coiling was safer than clipping in patients with an aneurysm 10 mm or less in diameter and with a favorable shape for coiling. This finding was true even though coiling was associated with a higher rate of postoperative rebleeding than clipping. Again, this finding should not be interpreted to mean that "coiling is safer than clipping for all brain aneurysms," particularly given that significant flaws have been identified in the International Subarachnoid Aneurysm Trial (**Chapter 24**).

Although the International Subarachnoid Aneurysm Trial is an important trial, the public should be aware of the potential for misinterpreted conclusions and methodology from third parties. There is always a potential for self-interest groups to present data, or portions of data, in a self-serving manner. Furthermore, coiling is also associated with complications, some of which are serious and life-threatening (**Chapters 13** and **18**). Complications related to coiling may still be underreported. As more studies are conducted, the short- and long-term safety and efficacy of coiling compared with those of open surgery for the treatment of brain aneurysms will eventually be established. At present, these two main alternatives require careful and balanced consideration before a patient chooses which treatment to pursue.

A patient with a brain aneurysm who is older than 65 years or who has multiple medical problems such as significant heart or lung disease may be counseled toward coiling rather than clipping. Coiling seldom requires general anesthesia or prolonged hospitalization. For such patients, it may be safer as the first treatment consideration.

CHAPTER 13.

Informed consent

Informed consent is the process by which the physician communicates relevant and accurate information to the patient and his or her family members before performing a procedure. The process is not a one-way communication; rather, questions and concerns of the patient and family members can and should be addressed.

The treating cerebrovascular surgeon or endovascular surgeon should be expected to obtain informed consent from an aneurysm patient before proceeding with surgical or endovascular treatment. During the investigation and treatment of an aneurysm, a patient may encounter other procedures that require informed consent, including, but not limited to, cerebral angiography; lumbar puncture; and placement of an external ventricular drain, lumbar drain, or CSF shunt. The patient or family members may be asked to enroll in a relevant clinical trial or study. Such enrollment also requires that informed consent be obtained.

Informed consent should include an honest and candid discussion of the risks and expected benefits of the procedure. At the end of this discussion, a patient should be able to clearly weigh whether a procedure's benefits outweigh its risks, which is the usual expectation. Another topic that should be discussed in a comprehensive informed consent is appropriate alternative(s) to the proposed procedure, for example, observation of the aneurysm versus surgery versus endovascular treatment, or coiling the aneurysm alone versus coiling and stenting its parent artery, and so forth. Informed consent should indicate a team approach. A neurosurgeon-in-training, that is, a neurosurgical resident, chief resident, registrar, or a cerebrovascular fellow may assist the attending surgeon. Finally, informed consent for surgery or endovascular treatment should include a question by the doctor regarding the patient's "advance directives." That is, does the patient have a will or other written directive that informs the health care team and family members about the patient's wishes should he or she, at some point, become unable to communicate those wishes? The physician should document the patient's or family's response to all these questions and issues. A final statement regarding the patient's desires for care and the family members' agreement to proceed with the discussed procedure should also be documented.

In summary, a comprehensive informed consent includes a discussion of the following seven elements: (i) benefits and (ii) risks of the procedure, (iii) alternatives to the procedure, (iv) team approach, (v) advanced directives, (vi) the anticipated type and date of the procedure, and (vii) the desire to proceed as discussed.

In certain situations, a patient cannot provide informed consent, for example, a minor who is not legally an adult, which is typically defined as 18 years old. In the case of minors, the parents should be able to provide informed consent. Alternatively, a patient may have a significant cognitive or mental impairment, that is, he or she may be confused, comatose, demented, or significantly mentally challenged. The hospital facility should have guidelines about how to obtain consent in these special circumstances and about the type of care deemed medically necessary and in the best interests of the patient. Sometimes a hospital may receive a comatose patient with a ruptured aneurysm in need of a potentially life-saving procedure. If the medical personnel are unable to contact the patient's family members in such a life-threatening emergency and no advance directives are on record, the best interests of the patient should be the only consideration. In such a circumstance, physicians will typically act accordingly and attempt to do what they were trained to do: heal the sick and save lives.

The benefits and risks of procedures used to care for aneurysm patients are detailed below. Note that the following examples reflect guidelines. Percentages vary depending on the many factors discussed in **Chapter 11**. A patient and his or her family should discuss these issues with the treating physicians.

Cerebral catheter angiography. The main benefit of cerebral angiography is that it provides the most detailed look at the blood vessels of the brain. Metal clips and coils from previous clipping or coiling of an aneurysm can interfere with the signal obtained during MRI or MRA. Therefore, regular catheter angiography remains superior for follow-up imaging. The risks include about a 1% chance of stroke or vessel hemorrhage during the procedure, and a 1 to 2% chance of a local infection, blood clot, or formation of a peripheral aneurysm at the site of catheter puncture itself, that is, the femoral artery in the groin.

Aneurysm coiling and stenting. The benefits of this form of aneurysm treatment include no open surgery. Hospital stays are shorter and the risk of neurological impairment soon after treatment is less than with surgery. This form of treatment also may be better than open surgery in older patients, particularly those with significant medical problems. The risks of this form of aneurysm treatment include a 5 to 10% chance of complications during the procedure. The main problems are vessel injury or aneurysmal rupture and stroke. Other risks include incomplete treatment of the aneurysm and its recurrence after the procedure. Either of these latter risks will likely entail further treatment by repeat coiling or open surgery. The chance of an aneurysm recurring increases as the size of the aneurysm being coiled or stented increases.

Aneurysm surgery. The main benefit of aneurysm surgery is that it is usually curative. If the aneurysm is considered unsuitable for coiling, aneurysm surgery may be the only viable option. In such cases, the benefit of treating the aneurysm should outweigh the risks of observing it. If a surgeon believes that he or she has successfully clipped a brain aneurysm, the chance of it recurring is extremely low. Regardless of treatment, however, new aneurysms can occur at different locations. The percentage or chance of a complication with surgery may be as low as 5% but varies according to the multiple factors discussed in **Chapters 11** and **12**.

Complications of surgery include, but are not limited to, new neurological impairment such as confusion or new weakness, hemorrhage or infection involving the operative site, new seizures, and a very small chance of death under anesthesia. Any complication a person can think of can occur during surgery, but the chances of such complications occurring are usually low. Of course, despite the best efforts of the surgeon, an aneurysm may not be treated completely and may require further attempts at treatment via coiling or repeat open surgery.

External ventricular drainage. The main benefit of placing an external ventricular drain (**Chapter 7**) after SAH is to clear the ventricular system of blood to prevent hydrocephalus. An external ventricular drain also allows the pressure inside the brain, or ICP, to be monitored. If ICP rises, the neurosurgeon can remove CSF via the external ventricular drain to compensate for the increase. External ventricular drains are usually placed in the emergency room or ICU. The main risks are a 1 to 2% chance of brain hemorrhage during placement of the drain and a 1 to 2% chance of infection. An infection may be a superficial wound infection or a deeper infection such as ventriculitis or meningoencephalitis. To prevent infections, antibiotics may be administered intravenously around the time of external ventricular drain placement. The external ventricular drain tubing itself also may be impregnated with antibiotics before it is placed. Periodically, CSF from the external ventricular drain is collected and sent to the laboratory for analysis.

Lumbar drain placement and lumbar puncture. After an external ventricular drain has been removed, a lumbar drain (**Chapter 7**) may be placed to allow blood mixed with CSF to continue to be drained from a fresh site in patients still unable to absorb the CSF that they produce. Placement of a lumbar drain may represent a final attempt by the neurosurgical team to divert the CSF enough to avoid placement of a shunt. A lumbar puncture (**Chapter 7**) may be performed if the neurologist or neurosurgeon needs to determine if blood is present in the CSF of a patient whose history is suggestive of aneurysmal SAH, but whose CT scan shows little supporting evidence. Risks associated with lumbar puncture and placement of a lumbar drain include a 1 to 2% chance of infection, referred to as meningitis; hemorrhage; and a very small risk of leg paralysis. The risks of hemorrhage and paralysis may be higher in patients taking anti-platelet medications such as Aspirin, Ticlid, or Plavix, or in those taking anticoagulant medications such as Coumadin or Warfarin. The procedure may cause some pain from local electrical stimulation, pressure, or irritation of a nerve root. A local anesthetic is administered through the skin to make the procedure as painless as possible.

Shunt placement. Patients with a ruptured aneurysm who cannot be successfully weaned from an external ventricular drain or lumbar drain (**Chapter 7**) must have a shunt placed to treat their hydrocephalus. A shunt also allows patients to be mobilized, that is, to get out of bed and, it is hoped, to be released from the hospital sooner. The associated risks with shunt placement include a 10% chance of an infection requiring removal and replacement of the shunt hardware, a 10% chance of failure due to disruption or blockage of the tubing, and a 1 to 2% chance of hemorrhage in the brain or injury to the bowel during shunt placement. The symptoms and signs of shunt infection usually manifest within the first few weeks of shunt placement, but they also may appear later. Symptoms can include unexplained fevers, redness along the site of the shunt tubing, headaches, nausea, vomiting, blurred vision, neck stiffness, increasing sleepiness, and sometimes increasing abdominal pain and tenderness.

CHAPTER 14.
The perioperative period and the operation itself

The perioperative period refers to the few days before and after open surgery. Preoperative refers to the time before surgery, while the postoperative period refers to the time after surgery. Preoperatively, a patient should have met the microneurosurgeon who will perform the surgery. The discussion between patient and surgeon should have included some of the topics covered in the preceding chapters. The surgeon should have discussed the benefits, risks, alternatives, and team approach for surgery (Chapter 13); reviewed the basics of the surgery and recovery period, and addressed any of the patient's questions or concerns.

The patient also may have met a member of the anesthesia team involved in administering a general anesthetic to the patient and looking after the patient during the operation. The anesthesiologist will want to know the patient's basic medical history, medications, allergies, any previous experiences with anesthetics, and so forth.

For elective aneurysm surgery, that is, patients with unruptured aneurysms, a patient may have to undergo routine blood tests, chest radiographs, and electrocardiography to be formally cleared for surgery. Any further testing and consultation depend on the patient's medical condition, but the preoperative evaluation is fairly straightforward and brief for most patients. Patients should inform their doctor if they are taking medications that can thin the blood such as Coumadin, Warfarin, Plavix, Ticlid, and Aspirin.

The evening before surgery, a patient should have a good meal and get some rest. After midnight that night, the patient should not eat or drink anything. However, a patient should check with the doctor about taking any regular medications. On the morning of surgery, the patient arrives at the admitting area of the hospital. The check-in time for elective aneurysm surgery is usually early, because most neurosurgeons prefer that their elective brain aneurysm patients be their "first case." The admitting staff assists patients and their families. Typically, they confirm a patient's identity, the side on which the operation is to be performed (left or right), and answer any questions or concerns before surgery.

Most aneurysm surgeries take 3 to 5 hours of operating time. However, by the time a patient has been called for surgery, administered general anesthesia, operated on, awakened after surgery, observed in the postoperative recovery area, and transferred to the ICU, many more hours may pass. It is normal for family members to be anxious when a loved one is undergoing surgery, and there is usually a waiting area in the ICU or near the operating room complex for family members. If family members leave that area, they should leave a contact number with the staff there so that they can be reached, even if only for an update regarding how the surgery is proceeding. However, not all institutions have Communicators who provide such periodic updates during the surgery. Some aneurysm surgeries take longer to perform than others because of the complexity of the aneurysm or because more than one aneurysm is being treated. Before elective surgery, the neurosurgeon usually discusses this issue. A neurosurgeon will take "as long as it takes" to perform the surgery as skillfully and as safely as possible. When the surgeon is completed, the neurosurgeon or a member of the operating team usually speaks with the family personally to tell them how the procedure went and what to expect in the short term. If they have any concerns, family members should feel free to check with the desk staff.

For elective aneurysm surgery, the patient is usually brought to the operating room awake and oriented. One or more intravenous lines are placed if they were not already inserted in the preoperative or holding area. After the lines are placed, the patient breathes oxygen and anesthetic gases and is given intravenous sedation. In this manner the patient is safely and comfortably put to sleep and intubated. Intubation involves placement of a breathing tube, usually through the mouth and into the trachea, so that ventilation (breathing) can be controlled during the procedure when the patient will be under deep anesthesia.

Next, other lines are placed by the anesthesia team. An intraarterial line is placed in the wrist artery for continuous monitoring of blood pressure during the case. A deep intravenous line called a central line also may be placed to monitor the patient's cardiovascular system. Thereafter, the neurosurgical team gets involved.

The patient's head is appropriately positioned for the surgery. The body is well padded and secured to the operating room table. During surgery the head is usually held in place by a pinion. A pinion is a metal clamp with three points that are pushed through the skin of the scalp and pressure-adjusted to contact the outer bone of the skull. The pinion, which keeps the head very still during surgery, is removed at the end of the procedure. After the pinion is removed, the three pin holes are often filled with an antibiotic ointment. In most patients the holes seal on their own within 24 hours of surgery. The pin sites pose little significant risk of infection or cosmetic damage. They are very small and usually behind the hairline. Occasionally, one pin site is located in the forehead, but it should also heal well.

After the patient is positioned, the scalp hair is shaved. The degree of head shaving depends on the surgeon's preference. Many surgeons prefer a minimal head shave. That is, a 1 to 2 cm or a half-inch wide strip of hair shaved in the appropriate location, typically behind the natural hair line. Compared with a more extensive head shave, a strip shave is cosmetically appealing to most patients. Furthermore, there are no apparent disadvantages associated with a strip shave. There is no evidence of an increased risk of infection if usual aseptic (sterile) measures are followed. Once the surgical field is prepared with the appropriate antiseptic solutions and draped in a sterile manner, the operating room scrub staff prepare the equipment and surgery begins.

The scalp is incised with a scalpel. The cut flap of scalp is turned to provide good exposure of the cranial bone or "craniotomy site." The location of the craniotomy depends on the aneurysm. Frontotemporal or pterional craniotomies frequently involve the front and side of the head. As part of an orbitozygomatic approach, bones around the eye, cheek, or both may be removed but are replaced at the end of the procedure. The incision for the frontotemporal craniotomy or one its variants starts from just in front of the ear and proceeds upward and immediately behind the forehead hairline. It may swing slightly across the midline to the other side just behind the hairline. Another common craniotomy for an aneurysm located low in the posterior circulation is located toward the back of the head, namely, a lateral suboccipital craniotomy. The incision for the suboccipital craniotomy is curvilinear behind the ear.

After the scalp flap is turned, the exposed bone flap is removed using a high-speed drill. Small bur holes are made in the skull. With an appropriate attachment to seat the drill, the bone flap is turned. The exposed leathery covering of the brain, known as the dura, is then opened sharply with a scalpel and dural scissors. Once the dura is reflected out of the way, the surface of the brain can be seen. The operating microscope is brought into the field. The neurosurgeon meticulously defines the arteries around the aneurysm and then clips the neck of the aneurysm.

At the conclusion of the procedure, when the surgical field is dry, the dura is reapproximated with sutures. The bone flap is replaced and typically affixed with microtitanium plates and screws. It is restored so that a good cosmetic and structural result is obtained. Finally, the scalp is closed with multiple layers of buried suture. Either sutures or staples are used to close the skin.

After surgery the patient is transferred to the busy environment of the ICU. Most ICUs have waiting areas for family members. Most have numerous medical and paramedical staff members. The number of rooms varies. Some have only one room for one patient; others accommodate two or more patients. Each ICU room has a lot of medical equipment with lighted displays and sounds. Patients and family members should not be alarmed by these devices. The most obvious may be the monitor, which displays the vital signs such as heart rate and rhythm, blood pressure, blood oxygen level, and so forth. A stand for an intravenous line is present to hold the main intravenous fluid as well as pain and other medications. Some patients need a ventilator machine for the breathing tube. A thin plastic drainage tubing may be connected from the patient's head or back to a nearby stand as part of the external ventricular drainage or lumbar drainage system (**Chapters 7** and **13**). The patient's head may be wrapped. The wrap, which looks like a white gauze turban with or without a fishnet outer wrap, is a bandage that applies pressure around the head incision. Drainage tubing exits from the wrap and is connected to a drain left under the scalp to drain blood that can accumulate beneath the edges of the incision. If the wrap and drain are present, they are usually removed the day after surgery. Some surgeons leave no head wrap on the patient, while others leave a head wrap for 24 to 48 hours. The practice varies based on the surgeon's preference.

Some patients return to the ICU without a breathing tube. In such cases, the anesthesiologist believes that the patient met all requirements for extubation, that is, removal of the endotracheal tube after surgery. At the end of surgery the patient probably demonstrated that he or she was able to follow commands by appropriately squeezing hands and wiggling toes, and was awake and strong enough to manage his or her own airway without need for further assistance with a tube.

To some degree a breathing tube irritates the throat. For a few days after extubation, a patient may cough or spit up blood-tinged saliva. During this period, the patient also may have a dry or sore throat, which can usually be treated with humidified air and throat lozenges.

Within a few hours of surgery, extubated patients are lucid or awake enough to talk and interact relatively well. They still may be drowsy and in some pain. After the first night, the drowsiness usually subsides on its own accord. The head pain subsides with appropriate pain medication. If the patient seems to be in pain that is not being controlled appropriately, the nursing and medical staff may alter the medications or request a Pain Service specialist to assist in the patient's treatment. The first 7 to 10 days after surgery, patients usually experience pain from the incision or operation. The pain can usually be controlled with narcotic medications, which are first given intravenously and then orally. The pain then usually begins to subside. Typically, patients are asked to wean themselves from the oral pain medications within 7 to 14 days of surgery.

The ICU staff doctors include a neurologist, an anesthesiologist, or both with a special interest in critical care, and a neurosurgeon or neurosurgical resident or registrar. These doctors regularly check on their ICU patients who are also under close supervision by the ICU nursing staff. The nursing staff perform and chart the neurological status and vital signs of the patient. They also perform other routine but very important aspects of care, including administering pain medication, fluids, and food; positioning the patient; and caring for the patient's hygiene. Nurses inform doctors of any significant neurological changes in the patient's status. Other paramedical staff may manage the ventilator and urinary catheter if the patient is still dependent on such equipment. The doctors and nurses make every attempt to update families daily. At most centers, doctors visit their ICU patients at least twice daily. If patients or family members feel that they are not receiving enough reasonable updates or that their concerns are not being addressed, they should discuss their concerns with the nursing or medical staff or with the nurse manager of the ICU.

Patients may return to the ICU with an endotracheal tube for many reasons. A patient whose aneurysm ruptured before surgery may have already been in poor neurological condition. The recovery of such patients can be expected to be slow. SAH patients may need more time than patients with unruptured aneurysms before they are alert and strong enough to be extubated safely. Alternatively, the surgery may have been expectedly or unexpectedly complex. In such cases the surgeon and anesthesiologist may favor keeping the patient intubated the first night or so after surgery. In patients with aneurysms that ruptured near the brainstem, safe extubation may be hampered by swelling or injury of the lower brainstem pathways and nerves, some of which are closely involved with respiration, speech, and swallowing. Such patients may need a longer period of intubation to assist their breathing. Intubation also prevents them from inhaling swallowed substances, including saliva, into their lungs. This problem is referred to as aspiration. The doctors should provide information about these matters and their reasoning for prolonging intubation (**Chapter 17**). Overall, however, most patients with an unruptured aneurysm are successfully extubated at the end of surgery.

The early postoperative period, that is, within 24 to 72 hours of surgery, may involve the following scenarios in patients with unruptured aneurysms treated by open surgery. Although patients still may be drowsy, most are awake and talking on the night of surgery. Most spend the first night in bed rest, with a Foley or urinary catheter and intravenous fluids and medications to help them. The next day, most of these patients are encouraged to sit out of bed and to begin eating. The earlier patients get out of bed, the better it is for their lungs. Otherwise, the lungs of immobile or nonambulatory patients experience some degree of collapse and congestion. Being ambulatory is also good for the circulation; it helps to prevent blood clots in the legs and lungs.

Within 24 hours of surgery, most patients with an unruptured aneurysm should be expected to be walking again. After one night most move from the ICU to a bed in a regular ward or floor. Many are discharged from the hospital after 2 or 3 nights. Few require any specific physical therapy; rather, they are encouraged to walk as much as possible. Climbing stairs is encouraged, as are eating a nutritious, well-balanced diet and gradually resuming regular activities, including driving, sex, physical exercise, and work when their bodies tell them they are ready.

Hospital discharge criteria include being able to walk safely and independently, to eat, to excrete; having minimal or at least well-controlled pain; and a clean, dry, and intact incision. At discharge, the medical team should provide patients with a written summary of their stay and operation and a telephone number to call if they develop any concerns about their neurological condition, wound, or any other issues. Before leaving the hospital, the patient and family should be sure that they have such contact information. Patients should check with their neurosurgeon or medical team regarding postoperative follow-up visits. Many centers automatically mail this appointment information to patients. The timing of the visit varies from patient to patient and from surgeon to surgeon. However, appropriate follow up for all aneurysm patients is essential.

At discharge patients usually have staples or sutures in their incision. The patient's local doctor or nurse needs to check and remove these stitches at the appropriate time, typically 10 to 12 days after surgery. Suture or staple removal is not a painful procedure. Patients may feel a slight tugging, but there should be no significant discomfort. Alternatively, the patient's surgeon or his or her assistant can also remove the stitches according to the arrangements made at discharge. Overall, it takes 3 to 6 weeks from surgery for patients with an unruptured aneurysm to feel that they have recovered enough to resume a relatively normal life.

The early postoperative period of patients with a ruptured aneurysm may be different than the above description. The course of patients heavily depends on their neurological condition or "grade" at the time of their hospital admission after SAH. First, these patients may require prolonged intubation or a prolonged stay in the ICU. Second, it often takes longer to mobilize these patients because their brains have to heal from the effects of having blood where it does not belong. As a result, several days or longer may be needed before they are well enough to be moved out of bed safely, to walk, and to be disconnected from all their drips, lines, and tubes. They may have an external ventricular drain or lumbar drain and need to be monitored and treated for the development of vasospasm, sodium and fluid imbalances, and hydrocephalus (**Chapters 7** and **13**). Physical Medicine and Rehabilitation services (**Chapter 20**) may be consulted to help meet the physical needs of such patients to optimize their overall recovery. Patients may need only brief bedside physical therapy. Alternatively, at some point during their hospital stay, SAH patients may need to undergo inpatient rehabilitation to maximize their chance of attaining an acceptable physical recovery (**Chapter 20**).

CHAPTER 15.

The peri-interventional period and the procedure itself

Just as for the perioperative period, the peri-interventional period refers to the few days before and after endovascular treatment of the aneurysm. The endovascular surgeon meets with the patient to discuss the benefits, risks, alternatives, team approach, technical aspects of endovascular surgery, and the recovery period. An anesthesiologist may meet with the patient to ensure that he or she is medically cleared for the procedure, even if neither open surgery nor deep anesthesia is required. The endovascular surgeon may recommend that the patient be placed on a blood thinner such as Plavix for the procedure. Having the patient take a blood thinner before platinum microcoils, stents, or both are placed prevents the parent artery feeding the aneurysm from suddenly blocking off or thrombosing, which can cause a stroke. Microcoils and stents are intrinsically thrombogenic, that is, they slow blood flow around them enough to cause blood to clot. Through this process they "seal off" aneurysms. The endovascular surgeon informs the patient if blood thinner is needed before the procedure. If recommended, the load is usually administered as an oral medication the night before the procedure. Sometimes, however, the blood thinner is administered as an oral or intravenous medication at the time of the procedure.

As for surgery, the patient eats and drinks nothing after midnight the night before the procedure and checks with the doctor about whether any of the patient's regular medications should be taken. Most endovascular surgeons prefer to perform such procedures earlier in the day rather than later. The patient reports to the registration area of the hospital at the specified time and is directed to the angiography suite in which the procedure will be performed.

Typically, endovascular treatment causes no pain. Furthermore, a patient with an unruptured aneurysm seldom requires deep or general anesthesia. Instead, a modified anesthesia routine is used. Oxygen is administered via face mask or nasal cannula, and mild intravenous sedating medications are used to make the patient drowsy and settled but still somewhat cooperative. Local anesthetic is administered at the entry site of the catheter, typically in the groin. The thin catheter tubing is advanced painlessly through the aorta and into the arteries of the neck and brain. When contrast dye is injected into the patient's circulation through the catheter, the patient may feel a warm rushing sensation. There should be no other significant discomfort.

As the dye is injected, the radiograph machines rapidly take multiple radiographs and form a roadmap of the patient's brain circulation. The aneurysm is identified, and the microcoils, stent, or both are introduced or deployed through the catheter into the aneurysm. In the best-case scenarios, the aneurysm is then occluded completely and without complication. The devices are withdrawn, and manual pressure is placed on the femoral "puncture" site for 20 to 30 minutes to allow a suitable clot to form. An arterial closing device may be used instead.

The endovascular procedure itself may take 1 to 3 hours to perform. Additional time may be needed for anesthesia and recovery after the procedure. The patient may be kept flat in bed 4 to 6 hours after the catheter is removed to allow the femoral clot to form, so that no hemorrhage occurs at or from this site. A hemorrhage at this site is usually marked by an expanding and often painful thigh clot. The patient should report any such signs to the nursing staff. The nursing staff also should be checking for a clot on a regular basis after the patient returns to the recovery room and in the ICU.

Most patients who undergo endovascular treatment of an unruptured aneurysm spend one night in the ICU. Most of these patients are discharged from the ICU directly to home the next morning. There are two exceptions: patients with a ruptured aneurysm, whose postprocedural care is the same as described for surgical patients in **Chapter 14,** and patients who suffer a complication during the endovascular procedure. For patients with an unruptured aneurysm who have undergone uncomplicated coiling, the night of the procedure is usually unremarkable. They should be awake, talking, and appropriately interactive soon after the procedure. After a brief period of bed rest, they are frequently encouraged to sit in a chair.

Patients should experience little pain. Some degree of headache is common after aneurysm coiling, particularly following coiling of basilar artery aneurysms. Patients also may have a minor aching pain in the thigh caused by the puncture. The endovascular surgeon should make recommendations regarding the treatment of the headache, which usually involves oral medications for a few days. If it occurs at all, this dull or throbbing headache usually subsides within a few days. It is not like the severe thunderclap headache associated with aneurysmal SAH. If the latter happens any time after the procedure, the patient should immediately seek medical attention. Sometimes higher doses of a nonsteroidal inflammatory medications such as Motrin, Advil, or ibuprofen can be used regularly for a few days till the headache subsides. However, patients should check with their endovascular surgeon before taking these medications.

On the day of discharge, usually the day after the procedure, patients should be given clear contact and follow-up instructions. If patients do not receive such information, they should check with their physician and nursing care givers. After endovascular treatment of an aneurysm, patients must return for follow-up evaluation because an aneurysm can recur or regrow. Future angiograms should be scheduled and the dates communicated to patients before they leave the hospital.

CHAPTER 16.
Wound issues

Wound healing is an important aspect of surgery and recovery. Healing can be impaired by preexisting medical problems such as diabetes mellitus, poor nutrition, poor levels of activity, smoking, and chronic use of steroids or nonsteroidal anti-inflammatory medications such as ibuprofen and Aspirin. Conversely, a good balanced diet, regular walking, and multivitamins are likely to be of benefit. There are other causes of wound problems. Eyeglass frames can continually rub over or scratch the incision. For eyeglass wearers undergoing a frontotemporal craniotomy, a soft padded piece of gauze can be taped to the frames to buffer between the incision and the plastic or metal frame near the ear. This padding should be worn for a few days after the sutures or staples are removed, that is, about 2 weeks.

Surgical wounds should be treated with respect. Many surgeons permit patients to shower some time the day after surgery. The wound does not need to be covered during a shower, but no shower spray should be applied directly to the incision. It is acceptable for water to run over the incision. At the end of the shower, the incision should be dabbed dry gently, not rubbed or abraded. Patients should avoid shampooing their hair the first 48 hours after surgery. Thereafter, a baby shampoo can be used everywhere except directly on the incision. Creams, oils, or ointments should not be applied to the incision. It is best to let the incision air dry. Because dampness can breed infection, some neurosurgeons recommend that patients avoid a tub, spa, or swimming pool for 2 to 3 weeks after surgery. However, this recommendation varies among surgeons; therefore, patients should check with their surgeon first. A few days to a week after the staples or sutures have been removed, patients can begin normal showering, bathing, and shampooing as long as the incision is healing as expected.

Deep tissue takes weeks to a few months to heal well. Any signs of wound infection, as detailed below, should be reported to the doctor at once. Sutures and staples are removed 10 to 12 days after surgery. If the closure was subcuticular, that is, the sutures were buried under the skin, then Steri-strips (butterfly-like stickies) may have been applied to the surface of the skin instead. These strips need to be removed 7 to 10 days after surgery after the patient takes a shower. Leaving these strips in place longer than 7 to 10 days increases the buildup of grime and the chance of infection. New skin glues may be used instead of Steri-strips and skin staples or sutures. Within a week or two of application, such glues should dissolve on their own. Sutures and staples can be removed by the patient's local nurse or doctor or by the neurosurgeon or his or her assistant. Although there may be some gentle tugging, removing sutures or staples is not painful and requires no injection. Some neurosurgeons recommend a period of 24 hours shower-free after the sutures or staples are removed so that the tiny holes can seal.

Numerous issues can arise regarding the incision or the operative site. These issues are worth considering one by one:

Wound infection. Despite the best efforts of neurosurgeons and operating room personnel, 1 or 2 of every 100 craniotomy patients develop a wound infection. That is, the infection rate is 1 to 2%. There is a 1% chance of a wound infection developing at the groin puncture site for angiography or coiling. Many of these infections are superficial and require only a brief course of oral antibiotic therapy. Other infections, however, are deep. In such cases, the incision must be reopened, the infected tissue cleaned, and infected edges of the skin debrided. When applicable, the bone flap may need to be removed and discarded. In these rare cases, the bone flap may be replaced months later with a synthetic bone substitute or a titanium mesh. This procedure is known as a cranioplasty.

Wound infections are usually obvious 10 to 14 days after surgery. A small amount of redness and mild swelling near the incision is normal soon after open surgery. However, these signs should subside 5 to 6 days after surgery. If the wound is getting more red, swollen, "boggy," and tender 10 to 14 days after surgery or if it begins to drain blood-stained fluid or pus, the patient needs to seek medical attention at once. Unexplained fevers associated with headache, nausea, vomiting, neck stiffness, or confusion are signs that a deep infection may be involving the brain or its coverings.

Patients suspected of having a wound infection should be examined by their local doctor or neurosurgeon. The doctor can follow a patient's healing clinically by bedside examination, by certain blood tests, and by CT of the head. Most wound infections resolve with appropriate management. The few patients who require removal of their bone flap usually have a good outcome after undergoing a cranioplasty to restore the cosmetic and structural integrity of the operated region.

During the time that the bone flap is removed, no full-time helmet is required for adults. Rather, once patients return home to await future cranioplasty, they should exercise general precautions against falls and head injuries. During this period, for 2 months after cranioplasty, or as advised by the surgeon, patients should avoid bike riding, rollerblading, and contact sports.

CSF leakage. Leakage of clear tear-like fluid from an incision or other site is uncommon after aneurysm surgery but needs to be reported to the doctor should it occur. Depending on the surgical site, CSF also may leak from the ear, an event known as otorrhea, or from the nose, an event known as rhinorrhea. CSF rhinorrhea may manifest as a continuous salty taste down the back of the throat or as tear-like fluid dripping like a tap from the nose. CSF leaks from incisions can be treated by oversewing the wound in the physician's office or emergency room under local anesthetic. The wound should then be rechecked in an outpatient setting. Alternatively, a lumbar drain can be placed for a few days and a pressure head wrap applied while the patient is observed in a hospital inpatient setting. It is extremely rare for an aneurysm patient to require surgery for a CSF leak (exploration and revision of the wound) if hydrocephalus is not the cause of the leak. Hydrocephalus increases pressure in the brain and forces CSF out a path of least resistance, such as a fresh incision or the site of a previous external ventricular drain. To treat delayed hydrocephalus, which is uncommon but can occur in ruptured aneurysm patients, a shunt is usually placed.

Swelling. After surgery some swelling in the incision area is normal. Sometimes the swelling is dramatic and can even cause the eye on the same side of the surgery to swell shut for several days. Depending on the type of craniotomy, the affected eye may be bruised. The bruising can persist for several weeks before subsiding. For swelling around the wound, ice packs and walking can be helpful. If the swelling does not begin to subside within 3 to 5 days of surgery, the patient should contact his or her doctor.

Sometimes CSF or dissolving blood clot fluid collects under the scalp. Such a collection usually resolves by reabsorbing on its own after several days. However, if the collection under the scalp enlarges, it may be a sign that the patient has hydrocephalus, especially if the patient had a ruptured aneurysm. A CT scan of the head should be obtained. The CT also may rule out infection of the underlying deep scalp and skull bone as a cause of delayed swelling in a wound.

Cosmetic issues. Most craniotomy wounds heal well, and most lie behind the hair line and are invisible. However, some craniotomies can be complicated by cosmetic issues. For example, there may be loss of muscle bulk, referred to as atrophy, in the temporalis muscle. This muscle, which is at the side of the head in the temple or temporal region just in front of and above the ear, is involved with chewing. During a frontotemporal or pterional craniotomy for aneurysm clipping, the temporalis muscle is retracted and then reattached at the end of the procedure. A bone flap also can settle, and a ridge, microtitanium plate, or screw head can be felt under the skin. When weighing survival from an aneurysm against these cosmetic issues, patients and physicians alike tend to agree that these cosmetic nuisances are acceptable parts of surgery.

Pain, numbness, and dysesthesia. Patients experience pain after surgery because tissues must be incised to perform the operation. For most patients, the pain is well controlled with medications administered intravenously soon after surgery and converted to oral pain medications soon thereafter. For most patients, their pain is substantially better 2 to 4 days after surgery and almost resolved within 7 to 10 days. Pain medications are then weaned. The pain threshold for each patient varies, but most patients are pain free within 2 weeks of their operation. Persistent pain is uncommon and should be reported to the doctor.

Many patients report some form of isolated numbness or a strange feeling referred to as dysesthesia around some part of the incision. This sensation, which is likely caused by the cutting of small sensory nerves in the incision site, tends to resolve within weeks to months of surgery. Sometimes, however, it persists. Treatment is seldom sought or offered for this minor complication, which again, is usually acceptable compared to the life-threatening nature of an aneurysm.

Some patients report discomfort with chewing or are unable to open their mouth completely. This complication usually follows a frontotemporal or full orbitozygomatic craniotomy in which the temporalis muscle is incised early in the operation. It typically resolves as the incision heals, but it may take several days to several weeks. Physical therapy for the jaw is recommended for those rare patients whose symptoms persist. Finally, some patients undergoing a craniotomy report symptoms such as "fluid in the ear," "ear fullness," or a "crackling sound." These ear symptoms typically disappear within days to weeks. However, patients should report fluid dripping from the ear to their doctor.

CHAPTER 17.
The comatose patient

A comatose patient exhibits little or no spontaneous self-generated activity, apart from breathing, and is unresponsive or poorly responsive to the outside world. The care of a comatose patient is complex. Significant and meaningful recovery may be delayed by weeks to months. At times there may be no meaningful recovery. The medical team tends to be aggressive with the care of comatose patients, whenever such a stance is appropriate and potentially beneficial. The level of care offered may evolve according to the patient's progress over time. Any significant change in the level of care offered to a patient is only pursued after a thorough and informed discussion between the physician and the patient's family members to reach a mutually acceptable consensus.

There are many important aspects of the care of comatose patients.

Advance directive. An advance directive is some form of legal document such as a Living Will or a special hospital advance directive form signed and dated by a patient, licensed health care provider, and a witness. Alternatively, it may be a Health Care power of attorney plan. An advance directive provides direction to health care workers about the patient's desired level of care should the patient be unable to communicate or to provide health care directives. Such situations include coma or significant cognitive impairment from any cause after admission. It is important for patients to plan ahead by making an advance directive and to discuss it with their spouse, other family members, and doctor. In considering the following general points, a patient should be sure to obtain the up-to-date and location-specific recommendations that apply to him- or herself.

First, an advance directive can be changed or revoked by patients at any time. Cognitively unimpaired patients have the capacity and right to decide about the type of treatment that they want if certain critical circumstances arise. Life-sustaining treatments to consider include mechanical ventilation, dialysis, blood transfusion, antibiotic therapy, and artificial nutrition and hydration therapies.

Second, advanced directives may include a status such as "do-not-resuscitate" or "do-not-intubate" in the event of cardiorespiratory arrest, that is, when heart and/or lung function ceases, or if other major clinical decline renders the patient critically ill and unable to provide directives. A physician directly involved in a patient's care can write a do not resuscitate status for a comatose or seriously ill and severely incapacitated patient, but it should be discussed with family and colleagues and the appropriate consensus reached.

Third, a Living Will should clearly state the circumstances and details of health care that a patient does or does not wish to have. This document should be signed and dated by the patient and a notary. An appropriate notary is an independent person who is not a beneficiary of the patient's Will, and not his or her health care provider, power of attorney, guardian, surrogate, or next of kin. A Health Care power of attorney document should be signed and dated in a similar manner.

Finally, when considering advanced directives, the patient's wishes and best interests should always be put first. To the best of their abilities, physicians and family should try to determine "What would the patient have wanted or decided if able to make ongoing care decisions?" The preferences of the patient should prevail.

Chest percussion therapy. This treatment is provided by one or more respiratory therapists and nurses. Certain modern ICU beds also provide chest percussion therapy. Treatment involves clapping on a patient's chest to break up secretions that can build up after a comatose patient spends prolonged periods supine or lying down. Chest percussion therapy is an important part of preventing or minimizing collapse of the lungs, a condition referred to as atelectasis. Atelectasis is a breeding ground for inflammation and/or infection of the lungs, that is, pneumonitis or pneumonia.

Feeding and Nutrition. Comatose patients cannot eat voluntarily. As a result, a feeding tube, which is a thin, soft plastic tube, may be passed by a physician or nurse through the patient's nose into the stomach for feeding and for administering oral medication. After a few weeks, a general surgeon or gastroenterologist may convert this tube to a percutaneous gastrostomy (PEG) or percutaneous jejunostomy (PEJ). These devices are tubes directly inserted from the surface of the abdominal skin into the stomach or adjacent small intestine for long-term feeding. The type of feeding formula provided through either a feeding tube or a percutaneous gastrostomy or percutaneous jejunostomy varies according to the hospital's practices and recommendations of the Nutrition Service.

Ventilation and airway support. A comatose patient is unable to support their own airway safely and may be unable to generate enough airway pressure and volume to breathe effectively. In such circumstances, they are placed on mechanical ventilators or breathing machines until they no longer require the apparatus or until its use is discontinued. An endotracheal tube is used to keep the airway of a comatose patient open. If still needed after about one week, the endotracheal tube may be converted to a tracheostomy tube, or "trache." A tracheostomy is a short airway tube inserted directly through the throat into the windpipe. It is placed to prevent pressure-related injury from an endotracheal tube to the patient's airway tissue. For a patient with a tracheostomy tube to talk, the tube must be manually capped at the surface of the throat. When the patient recovers, the tracheostomy can be removed and the throat opening sutured close.

Repositioning and skin care. Changing a comatose patient's body position and vigilant monitoring of the patient's skin for signs of pressure-related injury are essential in preventing breakdown of the skin and infection. Such infection can even spread to the blood stream, a condition referred to as wound-related sepsis. Nurses and physical therapists are particularly attentive to this issue. Should pressure sores develop, they are treatable. However, the best treatment is prevention. Sometimes treatment requires the input of a nurse specialist in skin care or a plastic surgeon.

Toileting and hygiene. A comatose patient typically retains bowel and bladder function. The intravenous fluids are eventually excreted by the kidneys, out through the urethra, and into a catheter tube. Periodically, the catheter is changed to prevent infection, and urine samples are sent to the laboratory to evaluate for signs of infection. Comatose patients may defecate less frequently than normal and may do so directly onto bed sheets. Typically, clothing and linen are immediately changed by the nursing staff to prevent infection and to maintain optimal patient health and hygiene. Regular bed baths, including sponge baths, and hair and oral hygiene, are provided by nursing and paramedical staff. These tasks are also important in maintaining the dignity of comatose patients.

Bedside Physical Therapy. This topic is discussed in detail in **Chapter 20**.

Prevention of DVT and pulmonary embolism. DVTs are blood clots that develop, usually in a deep or major vein in the leg. Sometimes, they also develop in a deep arm vein. Such clots may develop because that limb is not working normally, spending most of the time lying dormant in a comatose patient, despite efforts of nursing staff and physical therapists. DVTs usually manifest with limb swelling in comatose patients, while awake patients often report an aching limb. Ultrasound of the limb usually confirms the presence of the clot.

The major risk of DVT is migration of clot fragments through the circulation to the lung. This event, referred to as pulmonary embolism, can be fatal. Treatment options that may be required after DVT or a pulmonary embolism include intravenous blood thinners if deemed safe enough to use. If there is no effective alternative to the use of blood thinners, a vena cava filter is placed. Such a filter is a small umbrella that collects clot material before it can reach the heart and lungs. To prevent DVT and pulmonary embolism, medical teams usually apply thigh or knee-high thromboembolic disease stockings to bedbound patients and order the use of sequential compression devices. The latter are automatically reinflating devices that squeeze the calf muscles to circulate blood in this region. The device attempts to minimize hemostasis or slowed blood circulation that otherwise promotes the development of DVT. Many doctors use subcutaneous shots of low-dose blood thinners, such as subcutaneous heparin, Fragmin, Lovenox, or some equivalent. Early mobilization of a patient is helpful but challenging if the patient is comatose.

CSF drainage. Issues related to the placement of external ventricular drains and lumbar drains are discussed in **Chapters 7** and **13**.

Disposition. This refers to the appropriate placement for comatose patients. Typically, it refers to their place in an ICU because their vital functions cannot be monitored and supported adequately in any other setting. However, when ICU status is no longer deemed effective or appropriate for comatose patients and is withdrawn after the appropriate discussions, disposition may then refer to a hospital ward, hospice, nursing home facility, or home. The choice depends on the patient's medical condition and other factors, including logistics such as bed availability and the family's resources. Disposition may be guided by the patient's medical condition and advanced directives, the family members' wishes, and the aid of nursing staff and a social worker.

Withdrawal of support. Withdrawal of support is an important consideration for patients who are deemed by both physicians and family members to be in such poor neurological condition that a meaningful recovery is unlikely. To withdraw support, patients' documented or perceived expectations under these conditions must be considered. Withdrawal of support means that all life-sustaining treatments, investigations, and supportive therapies will cease, including ventilator and supplemental oxygen support, blood and imaging tests, intravenous hydration, all medications other than pain medications, and all nutrition. Instead, physicians usually prescribe comfort care measures, including a regular dose of subcutaneous or intravenous pain medication such as morphine or fentanyl and humidified air to ensure comfortable breathing for the patient.

The goal of the withdrawal of support is to continue to relieve pain and suffering while providing and promoting dignity in the patient's last few hours or days. Withdrawal of support may hasten death. Physicians and family members alike must feel that the withdrawal of support is appropriate and must be based on adequate levels of informed communication between physicians and family members.

Sometimes institutional, that is, hospital-based, or judicial, that is, legal body-based, intervention is necessary. This situation can occur if no significant family member or surrogate is available, if a dispute occurs among significant family members in the absence of advanced directives, or if a doctor believes that there is a conflict between a family's interests and a patient's best interests in the absence of an advance directive. A hospital Ethics Service Consultation or Ethics Committee may be asked to provide input, but it is seldom legally binding. Rather, the committee serves more of an advisory role. Such a committee or service may include an independent doctor, nurse, Justice of the Peace, attorney, hospital administrator, social worker, and chaplain.

Caring for the caregiver. Although last in this chapter, this issue is by no means the least consideration. Being diagnosed with and treated for an unruptured or ruptured aneurysm is extremely stressful not only for the patient, but also for the patient's loved ones. Broken sleep, continuous worrying, and the alien environment and unfamiliar faces of a large hospital can take their toll on the physical and emotional health of the patient's loved ones. That is why, to the best of their ability, loved ones should maintain regular and healthy rest and nutrition practices. A patient's healing is closely related to the support of his or her family and social network. Therefore, the ongoing health and well-being of a patient's loved ones are important parts of the overall equation for healing and recovery.

CHAPTER 18.
Complications of treatment

No treatment option is free of the risk of complications. The risk of complications depends on many factors, including the size and location of the aneurysm, whether the aneurysm is unruptured or ruptured, the type of treatment available, the patient's age and general medical condition, and the microneurosurgeon's or endovascular surgeon's experience. Aneurysm regrowth after previous clipping or coiling may increase the risk of subsequent open surgery or endovascular treatment.

The complication rate associated with unruptured aneurysms treated by endovascular means or open surgery is low. This is particularly true of smaller aneurysms (< 10 mm) located in the anterior circulation, which includes the internal carotid artery and its branches such as the ophthalmic, posterior communicating, and anterior choroidal arteries; the middle cerebral artery; and the anterior cerebral and anterior communicating arteries. For such aneurysms, the overall chance of a significant neurological or medical complication should be less than or equal to 5%. That is, there is a 95% or better chance that open surgery or endovascular treatment will be performed without significant complication. For larger aneurysms, especially those 10 mm or greater in diameter, and for those located in the posterior circulation (that is, the vertebral artery, vertebrobasilar junction, basilar trunk, basilar artery apex, or posterior cerebral artery), the risks of surgery increase with the complexity of the aneurysm. Surgical complication rates may be higher for patients with a ruptured aneurysm regardless of its size or location because of the presence of a blood clot and the "stickiness of tissue," an unstable aneurysm wall, brain swelling, and trauma. Overall outcomes are influenced by the severity of the initial hemorrhage and by the patient's medical condition before treatment is offered.

What types of treatment complications can occur?

Certain types of treatment-related complications encountered by aneurysm patients are discussed in **Chapters 13** and **16**. A few additional general points need to be considered.

Certain complications apply to patients undergoing open surgery. Their treatment and postoperative care are usually more complex and prolonged compared with that of patients undergoing endovascular treatment. General medical complications among patients undergoing open surgery include death (< 1%) from a very rare reaction to anesthesia, deep venous thrombosis, and pulmonary embolism. After surgery, patients may develop the new onset of seizures, but they persist only days to a few months. A major stroke or other brain tissue injury can cause a permanent neurological disability such as impaired eyesight, double vision, speech and swallowing difficulty, facial and/or limb weakness or paralysis, incoordination, and imbalance. A more specific discussion of potential complications is deferred to a patient's treating physician.

After either endovascular or open surgical treatment, most patients with unruptured aneurysms fare well in the long term. In comparison, the poor outcomes of patients with ruptured aneurysms is not necessarily related to a treatment-specific complication. Rather, their poor outcomes are related to the brain injury caused by the hemorrhage. The rate of complications "quoted" to a patient by his or her endovascular surgeon or microneurosurgeon should be the physician's personal complication rate, rather than those reported in the literature, which may be higher or lower. Such rates depend on the numerous factors mentioned above.

CHAPTER 19.

Recurrent, persistent, or new aneurysm after treatment and the need for follow-up

A recurrent aneurysm is one that regrows after the endovascular surgeon or microneurosurgeon thought that the aneurysm was obliterated by the patient's treatment. A persistent aneurysm is one that continues to grow because the endovascular surgeon or microneurosurgeon was aware that it was not completely obliterated during the initial attempt at treatment.

There are several reasons why an aneurysm may not be obliterated completely. The neck of the aneurysm may have been too large or too awkward for the attempted treatment, or its shape may have been too complex. The microneurosurgeon or endovascular surgeon may have been forced to leave a portion of the aneurysm untreated by clip or coil, respectively, because of a critical artery at that point on the aneurysm that needed to be preserved. Finally, a new aneurysm is one that occurs at a different location than any other aneurysm that was known and treated.

After effective open surgical treatment, the chance of the same aneurysm recurring or regrowing is low. If an endovascular surgeon or microneurosurgeon could not fully obliterate the aneurysm, the chance of the same aneurysm growing is significantly higher. In such situations, the chance of detecting ongoing growth in that aneurysm is about 1% per year. For endovascular treatment of aneurysms with a diameter larger than 10 mm, the chance of the same aneurysm recurring or regrowing is between 25 and 50%. The actual risk depends on the aneurysm's original size, regardless of how well the endovascular treatment seemed to have gone. Of these aneurysms, about half can be effectively re-coiled. Those that cannot are frequently referred to microneurosurgeons for treatment.

If a patient has had a ruptured aneurysm and a new aneurysm is found on follow-up imaging, most physicians will likely recommend treatment, or at least following the lesion with imaging, regardless of its size. The chance of a patient developing multiple intracranial aneurysms is 20 to 30%. That is, at diagnosis about 1 in 4 patients have multiple brain aneurysms.

For all of the reasons discussed above, it is important that patients undergo appropriate clinical and radiological follow up after treatment of their aneurysm. Typically, the frequency of follow up visits for well-clipped aneurysms is less than that for aneurysms treated by endovascular means. Excellent long-term data are available for surgically clipped aneurysms. Given that the technology is relatively new and still evolving, outcome data on endovascularly treated aneurysms are still young,

For example, consider a patient diagnosed with a ruptured aneurysm. No other aneurysm is identified at the time of the patient's initial hospital admission. Further assume that the patient's aneurysm is clipped successfully and no remnant is seen on intraoperative or immediate postoperative cerebral angiography. In such cases, some neurosurgeons would obtain the next follow-up cerebral angiogram 3 years after surgery. If there was no regrowth and no other aneurysm was seen at that time, the next angiogram might be obtained 10 years after surgery. If again there was no regrowth and no other aneurysm, another angiogram might be obtained 20 years after surgery. If at any time, however, regrowth or a new aneurysm is detected, further investigation and treatment are deferred to the patient's physician.

CHAPTER 20.
Recovery and rehabilitation

The recovery period for elective treatment in patients with an unruptured aneurysm is usually shorter and less complex than that for emergency treatment in patients with a ruptured aneurysm. Physically and psychologically, aneurysmal SAH can take its toll on patients and family. Physically, patients undergoing open surgery may have wound-related discomfort (**Chapter 16**) and fatigue. Fatigue, which may be described as feeling drained or generally weak, can persist for a few months after hospitalization. It usually improves with time. Regular napping and eventually weaning off medications such as those for pain or seizures according to the physician's recommendations may help improve such fatigue. New physical impairment(s) after SAH include problems with balance and coordination, weakness in one or more limbs, difficulty with speech and swallowing, and problems with vision. Over time such deficits may improve partially or entirely. Physically, healing may take months to a few years, and patients may need physical therapy.

Psychologically, patients may have problems associated with depression, emotional or behavioral instability, or slowed or abnormal brain processing (referred to as cognitive dysfunction). Cognitive dysfunction also may include impairment of language and memory functions. All of these problems may negatively impact a patient's sexual functioning and sex drive. Again, these psychological and cognitive problems may take months or years to improve completely or partially.

Family members of a survivor of a ruptured brain aneurysm may need to make difficult decisions and deal with extremely challenging circumstances. It helps if they can remain strong, persistent, and united through this difficult time. The patient is likely facing a life-altering event. Recovery often requires considerable patience, ongoing love, and support. People who survive the rupture of a brain aneurysm frequently need more help than they were previously used to or more than they may be willing to accept. Such help is critical. It may be in the form of physical therapy; speech therapy; a psychologist or psychiatrist; a home nurse; a temporary stay in a skilled nursing facility, rehabilitation center or a nursing home; increased contact and support from family members and friends; or increased interaction with a priest, church, or an equivalent religious or spiritual person or group. Time and positivity are essential.

Recovery from SAH is influenced by many factors.

Clinical presentation. Perhaps the foremost factor is the manner of an aneurysm patient's presentation. Some patients are neurologically devastated from the time of rupture. Others are surprisingly well despite the rupture. Some may only have a headache from a leak. Others may have an unruptured aneurysm detected by intentional screening or by chance.

Experience. Other important factors involved in a patient's recovery are the experience of the physicians and paramedical staff and the resources of the hospital facility at which the patient is treated. When elective treatment of an incidentally discovered aneurysm is being considered, a patient or family should research the treating doctors' backgrounds. Referrals and the Internet are potential sources of information. Having the procedure performed in a large teaching center, if possible, may be in a patient's best interest. For patients with ruptured aneurysms, the quality of the hospital's rehabilitation service is also paramount. The rehabilitation team of doctors and therapists are responsible for optimizing a patient's recovery after the patient has been treated.

Psyche. Finally, how critical a patient's mindset is to healing can hardly be overstated. Part of a patient's role in recovery means staying focused on healing, being positive, maintaining a healthy and balanced diet, walking and exercising as allowed, continuing to meet with family and friends as regularly as possible, and meeting the patient's spiritual needs. Returning to work, when possible, is a wonderful milestone.

Will "alternative" therapies help a patient?

Alternative therapies are outside of mainstream treatments—they do not include surgical or rehabilitation therapy. Alternative therapies include yoga, acupuncture, massage therapy, and hydrotherapy. Today the divide between mainstream and alternative therapy is narrowing. Hydrotherapy, however, may be a part of a mainstream physical therapy program.

Do alternative therapies help? Yes, some people, including aneurysm patients, often find that these alternative therapies help in the healing process. Like any treatment, however, these therapies will not help everyone. Will they help a specific patient? The answer to this question is unknown until a patient tries one or more of the treatments. Will they hurt? They are very unlikely to hurt a person in any significant way. In summary, one or more of these alternative therapies performed in a professional and safe way by caring and appropriately trained individuals may benefit certain patients.

Rehabilitation

Most patients with an unruptured brain aneurysm and some patients with a ruptured aneurysm require no formal inpatient or outpatient rehabilitation. However, many patients with a ruptured aneurysm do need these services. Rehabilitation services are available at most teaching hospitals, usually as part of a Department or Division of Physical Medicine and Rehabilitation. Rehabilitation services represent an umbrella for many subdisciplines, and the rehabilitation team is composed of several members:

Physiatrists. These physicians have specialized in rehabilitation medicine and oversee the rehabilitation process for patients admitted to their Service.

Physical Therapists. These individuals have special training in activities, both passive and active, that improve a patient's coordination, strength, and balance. Physical therapists work on specific muscle group movements and exercises and on the patient as a whole. Some physical therapists also train certain patients in the use of wheel chairs and walkers.

Occupational therapists. These team members work on activities directly relevant to a patient's daily living such as bathing; toileting; dressing; navigating around the ward, through rooms simulating a home-like environment, or in and out of a car. Some occupational therapists train certain patients in how to navigate wheel chairs and walkers in a home environment. They engage patients in games and activities that focus on dexterity and concentration.

Speech therapists. These professionals assess an individual's speech and swallowing function, both at the bedside and in an imaging suite. X-ray techniques are used for the formal assessment of swallowing function. Dysphagia, aspiration, and laryngeal penetration are terms commonly used to indicate a swallowing impairment. Speech therapists focus on exercises intended to improve speech and swallowing function. These functions can be impaired, particularly by aneurysms involving the brainstem and lower cranial nerves.

Social workers. These individuals assess the social support networks of a patient. They provide information about community support services that may be of direct benefit to certain patients and help coordinate the services for patients. They assist in finding appropriate placement for patients who are ready to be dismissed from a hospital facility but are not yet ready to transition to a home environment. Placement may be in a nursing home, a skilled nursing facility, or an acute rehabilitation facility.

Psychologists. These team members are trained in addressing the psychological stresses and needs of patients and their significant others. Specifically, they may assist in depression and behavioral counseling and may provide important recovery strategies for patients with significant memory and cognitive impairment.

Rehabilitation nurses. These members of the nursing staff have a special interest in the well being of rehabilitation patients.

Rehabilitation admission coordinators. As the title suggests, these coordinators act as liaisons among hospital, insurance services, and patients in the assessment of the suitability of patients for inpatient rehabilitation. Many rehabilitation services have specific criteria that must be met for inpatient stay. Such criteria involve determining if patients are neurologically impaired enough to require inpatient rehabilitation. For example, patients requiring inpatient rehabilitation must be awake and interactive enough to participate meaningfully in a minimum of 3 hours of rehabilitation exercises and activities each day. Furthermore, the patient's insurance should cover inpatient rehabilitation. If not, the request for transfer to the rehabilitation unit can be denied. However, rehabilitation may still be permitted at a unit closer to the patient's home. Alternatively, special charitable funds may be available from the hospital, or the Physical Medicine and Rehabilitation and Neurosurgical Services may negotiate directly with an insurance company through the hospital to see if an appropriate arrangement can be made.

What can a patient expect regarding rehabilitation?

Bedside rehabilitation. Most patients with ruptured aneurysms will have bedside rehabilitation. Typically, it begins with assessment by a physiatrist, followed by direct involvement of physical therapists and occupational therapists. A speech therapist also may be involved. If a patient is comatose or semi-comatose, rehabilitation services are still consulted for two reasons. First, basic range of motion exercises are commenced early to prevent or minimize the loss of muscle bulk and the development of joint contractures from disuse. Second, from an early stage, Physical Medicine and Rehabilitation Service for a critically ill or neurologically impaired patient is helpful for future inpatient rehabilitation planning. Some services may determine that a patient is physically and cognitively sound enough not to require rehabilitation. Instead, they may ask for formal assessment by physical therapists and occupational therapists from the perspective of safety as a patient transitions to home. This process is referred to as a home safety assessment. For example, can the patient get out of bed to a chair or walk a reasonable distance without falling? Can the patient get into a bath tub, dress independently, navigate around a room steadily, climb stairs, and eat without assistance? These therapists provide valuable advice to patients about their needs at home, including the need for bath rails, ankle orthoses, walkers, wheelchairs, and so forth.

Inpatient rehabilitation. Many ruptured aneurysm patients undergo a period of inpatient rehabilitation. Typically, the service is provided at the facility at which they were admitted. Sometimes, however, rehabilitation is conducted at a facility closer to their homes. Once the neurosurgery service is satisfied that it has done everything it can for patients who are still significantly neurologically impaired, the consulting Physical Medicine and Rehabilitation Service is requested to assume primary care. Such patients are transferred to the Physical Medicine and Rehabilitation floor or unit in the hospital. On the unit, the team members of the Physical Medicine and Rehabilitation Service can interact with the patient in a closer and more personal manner. In this environment, patients have direct access to the various rehabilitation programs and resources. The inpatient stay in rehabilitation varies from patient to patient according to their physical, cognitive, and psychosocial needs. It is usually a minimum of one week and may last several weeks. Discharge from a rehabilitation facility usually is based on a determination that patients are strong, mentally sound, and safe enough to transition to their home environment. If not, patients may be discharged to another rehabilitation facility closer to home for ongoing needs. In some instances, patients may be transferred directly to a skilled nursing facility, to an assisted living environment, or to a nursing home depending on their condition and needs.

Outpatient rehabilitation. This service is for patients who have already completed or are in too good a neurologic condition for inpatient rehabilitation. Such patients meet with community physical therapists, typically near their home. After discharge, outpatient physical therapy sessions may be as frequent as once daily or as infrequent as once weekly. Instructions are usually provided in the discharge summary or in a specific referral letter from the hospital physiatrist. The duration of outpatient rehabilitation varies from patient to patient. It may last a few weeks or a few months. The primary doctor should reassess the patient within 3 months of surgery and make any further recommendations for ongoing physical therapy needs, if any. Many physical therapists in the community require a written prescription for their services. For ongoing outpatient physical therapy, most prefer some form of referral letter or discharge summary from the primary doctor or hospital service.

CHAPTER 21.
Other types of brain aneurysms

The preceding chapters concern saccular or berry aneurysms (**Chapter 3**), which account for most of the brain aneurysms that receive medical attention. However, other types of aneurysms, known as nonsaccular aneurysms, also can occur in the brain. Although much rarer than their saccular counterparts, nonsaccular aneurysms can still be problematic.

Fusiform and dolichoectatic aneurysms. Fusiform aneurysms lack a distinct neck. They represent a widening of a segment of an artery around the entire vessel rather than just arising from a side of an artery's wall. They can rupture but usually do not. These aneurysms are thought to arise from the build up of fatty streaks or plaques inside blood vessels. High fat diets and smoking may play a role in their formation, as may genetic factors. They can also develop after mechanical injury to the inner part of the blood vessel wall such as a dissection.

As these lesions grow, the entire vessel wall may become expanded or ectatic. When this expansion is considerable, they are referred to as dolichoectatic aneurysms. On imaging scans these lesions appear as long, wide, serpentine aneurysms. Their mass can compress surrounding structures such as the brainstem. Any fibrofatty thrombus that they contain can fracture, flow through the circulation to other regions of the brain, and cause a stroke.

Once these aneurysms become large, they are notoriously difficult to treat. In their early stages, that is, as smaller fusiform aneurysms, they may be followed periodically with CTA or MRA. If the fusiform aneurysm is symptomatic, for example, causing stroke-like "thromboembolic" symptoms, treatment is usually directed at modifying the risk factors. This process can involve improving diet and exercise, using medications to lower cholesterol and blood pressure, checking for and treating diabetes, and/or prescribing a blood thinner or anticlotting medication.

Open surgical and endovascular options are reserved for such aneurysms that are unresponsive to medical treatments. These options are frequently high risk. Treatment may involve some form of trapping the aneurysm or sacrificing its parent vessel, with or without an open surgical brain bypass graft. A brain bypass is similar to a heart bypass, where another vessel is harvested by the surgeon and sewn in place to allow blood to bypass the diseased segment.

Unfortunately, some dolichoectatic aneurysms cannot be treated effectively with current technologies. They may continue to grow. Despite attempts at treatment, such aneurysms may even rupture. If a lesion is causing stroke-like events, it may be acceptable for a patient to be on a blood thinner. However, if these aneurysms rupture while the patient is on a blood thinner, the rupture can be fatal. The surveillance and treatment of these aneurysms are complex and should be discussed in detail with the physician.

Vein of Galen aneurysms. Although referred to as aneurysms, these lesions are unique. Rather than an artery, a deep vein of the brain known as the vein of Galen or a developmentally equivalent vein becomes massively enlarged as part of its involvement with an arteriovenous fistula or AVM. Vein of Galen aneurysms are very rare and typically found in infants and toddlers. They may be associated with heart failure, hydrocephalus, vision problems, and mental retardation. Sometimes, they are referred to as a venous varix, akin to a large varicose vein of the leg. They are treated by endovascular means more than by open surgery. They are high-risk lesions to treat.

Mycotic or infectious aneurysms. Mycotic aneurysms are more correctly referred to as infectious aneurysms. They arise from the spread of infectious particles, usually bacteria, into brain arteries. The infectious organisms set up an inflammatory response in the part of the vessel wall in which they lodge. The inflammatory response leads to a weakening of the wall, which dilates like an aneurysm. These lesions tend to look like fusiform aneurysms in that the dilatation usually lacks an appreciable neck. They tend to occur in more distant parts of the brain arterial tree.

Fewer than 5% of all brain aneurysms are infectious. About 10% of patients with bacterial endocarditis develop an infectious brain aneurysm. Therefore, a history of rheumatic fever is a risk factor for the development of these entities. Endocarditis can occur spontaneously or in intravenous drug users. The organism is classically a Streptococcus such as *Strep. viridans*, but may be a Staphylococcus such as *Staph. aureus*. It also may be a gram-negative organism or a mixture of organisms.

About 20% of patients with infectious aneurysms experience a rupture from the aneurysm. The evaluation of these aneurysms includes blood cultures; echocardiography, which is a detailed ultrasound of the heart chambers; and cerebral angiography.

Treatment is frequently medical, that is, intravenous antibiotics. If the aneurysm has ruptured or continues to grow despite adequate antibiotic therapy, surgery is typically offered. Surgery may involve sacrifice of the portion of the vessel from which the aneurysm arose. These aneurysms have walls that are notoriously friable and without necks. Therefore, they are unfavorable for clipping. Surgery may also involve brain bypass grafting.

New infectious aneurysms can grow, even in patients whose bacterial endocarditis and other known infectious brain aneurysms have responded to intravenous antibiotic therapy. Therefore, periodic surveillance with some form of brain angiography is recommended.

Dissecting or pseudoaneurysms. A dissecting aneurysm arises when the inner lining of a blood vessel is disrupted by mechanical trauma or by some form of ongoing inflammation within the wall such as fibrofatty build up. In such cases, blood seeps between the damaged layers of the arterial wall and reaches the adventitia (**Chapter 2**). There, the blood may be contained in a pocket. The pocket, however, can enlarge and eventually rupture. Dissecting aneurysms are referred to as pseudoaneurysms because they are not contained within the complete wall of a blood vessel. Rather, only part of the wall or tissues surrounding the blood vessel is involved if the aneurysm has ruptured. Depending on their size, shape, location, and the need for brain bypass grafting, these lesions may be treated by open surgery or endovascular surgery.

Aneurysms associated with AVMs. An AVM is a site of abnormal connectivity between arteries and veins. It looks like a tangle of worms. The greatest concentration of vessels is in the central portion of the AVM, which is referred to as the nidus. The nidus is composed of abnormal blood vessels that are hybrids between true arteries and veins (**Figure 11**). AVMs are fed by one or several arteries and are drained by one or more major draining veins. These feeding and draining vessels may be unusually tortuous, winding like rivers. Their bore may be unusually large. AVMs can occur in the brain or along the spinal cord.

Because the vessels of AVMs are abnormal, they may leak or rupture. Hemorrhage is the main complication. Blood flow and pressure in the vessels of an AVM are unusually high and may lead to significant shunting of blood to and from the lesion. In an AVM, high-flow pressure combined with abnormal structure of a vessel wall can lead aneurysms to form on the arteries that feed the AVM. This is the parent artery. Aneurysms involving the parent artery are called pedicle aneurysms. Aneurysms within the AVMs itself are intranidal aneurysms (**Figure 11**). The latter also can rupture. About 6 to 7% of brain AVMs have aneurysms associated with them.

When AVMs rupture, some physicians think that these associated aneurysms may have ruptured. Nonetheless, the abnormal nonaneurysmal components of the AVM are also thought to be prone to rupture. About 75% of the aneurysms associated with AVMs are pedicle aneurysms; the remainder are intranidal. Interestingly, if the AVM is treated effectively, pedicle aneurysms can fade away or disappear entirely. This is seldom the case for intranidal aneurysms. Aneurysms associated with AVMs are treated or removed at the time that the AVM is treated. Treatment can include open surgery, endovascular surgery, or a combination of both.

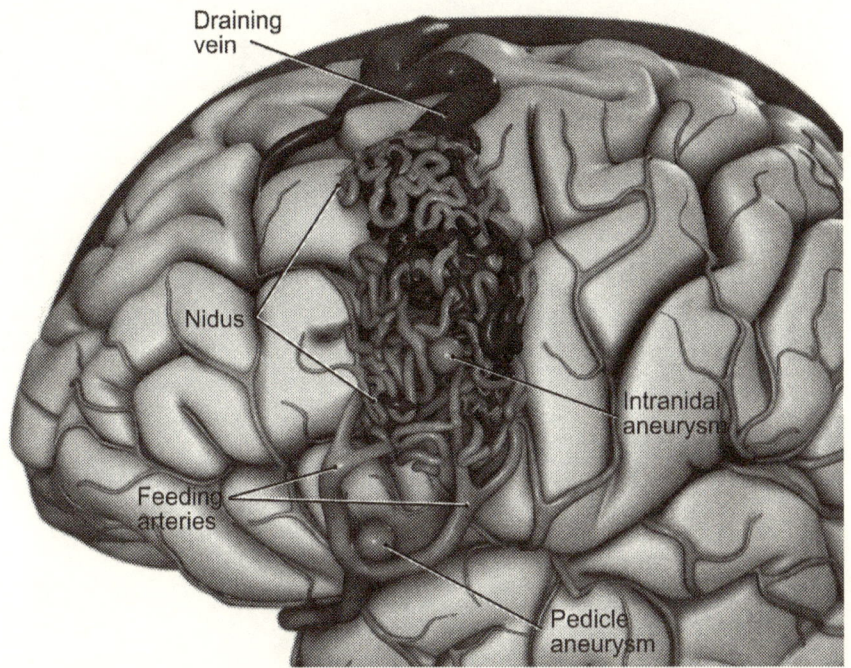

Figure 11. An AVM. The surface of the brain with an AVM originating there. The large and tortuous feeding arteries and draining veins can also be deeper in the substance of the AVM. The core or nidus of the AVM is located deep. The AVM usually forms a cone-shaped mass that extends from the pial or outermost surface of the brain down toward one of the ventricles. Note the possible presence of aneurysms on arteries feeding the AVM (pedicle aneurysm) or within the nidus itself (intranidal aneurysm). *With permission from Barrow Neurological Institute.*

CHAPTER 22.

The stories of four brain aneurysm patients

The stories of four patients with brain aneurysms follows. Pseudonyms have been used. The personal impact of aneurysmal disease on the two authors of this book is reflected by the fact that two of the patients in this account are relatives of the authors.

N.S.

On October 3, 1998, N.S., an otherwise healthy and active 42-year-old business executive and mother, experienced the worst headache of her life. She was at a luncheon with colleagues when she felt what she later described as a sudden pounding headache, like someone had struck her in the head with a baseball bat. The excruciating pain, which came without warning, moved rapidly from the right side of her head to all over. To the horror of her colleagues, she stood up holding her head, gagged, and then collapsed. She was still breathing when paramedics arrived, perhaps because one of her colleagues administered basic cardiopulmonary resuscitation in the interim. She was taken by ambulance to the closest teaching hospital and was unconscious throughout her journey. Finding her unconscious and fearing that she might stop breathing en route to the hospital, paramedics had placed a breathing tube at the scene.

On arrival in the emergency room, N.S. was pale and listless. Her blood pressure was high, and her breathing was supported by a ventilator. After a rapid clinical and neurological evaluation, she was taken to the CT scanner for a head scan. She was comatose but stable. Based on the history of a sudden, severe headache, it was suspected that she had a brain hemorrhage. Her gender, age, and history led her physicians to consider a ruptured brain aneurysm first, and a ruptured AVM second. No family members were available to describe her family history, and there was no record of her in the hospital's electronic charting system.

The findings on the CT scan suggested the presence of a brain aneurysm. Blood, which appears white on a CT scan, was present in many places where it should not have been present. The pattern indicated aneurysmal SAH. The team rapidly organized for N.S. to undergo cerebral angiography. While she was waiting for the angiogram, an external ventricular drain was placed in a fluid-filled cavity of her brain. The tube allowed some of the blood-mixed CSF to drain, which allowed her brain to relax a little. It also gave her neurosurgeons the ability to monitor her intracranial pressure. The angiogram showed a 7-mm aneurysm, with a daughter sac on its dome, located in the right middle cerebral artery. Blood clot surrounded the aneurysm, and her brain looked tight from swelling. Another small aneurysm (3 mm) was located in the left middle cerebral artery. It looked more uniformly round and less threatening than the other lesion. The remainder of the blood vessels in her brain looked normal.

The microneurosurgeon consulted his endovascular colleague to discuss how best to treat the two aneurysms and in what order. The right-sided aneurysm most likely had bled because the blood clot was thicker around this site and because this aneurysm was largest and ugliest. The goal was to obliterate the right-sided aneurysm from her brain circulation rapidly and completely to prevent it from rerupturing. If N.S. only had the aneurysm on the left and no history of rupture, some physicians might have elected to follow that aneurysm with periodic imaging. However, given that she had experienced a rupture, the surgeons thought that both aneurysms should be obliterated. They agreed that although the aneurysms could be coiled, the lesion on the right had a wide neck and other features that made it less likely to be completely obliterated by coiling. Nonetheless, the consensus was to attempt coiling. Furthermore, she was already in the angiography suite.

The endovascular surgeon first attempted to treat the left-sided aneurysm, which looked less threatening. Two platinum microcoils were placed within it. At the end of this part of the procedure, the lesion appeared to be obliterated completely. He then turned his attention to the aneurysm on the right. Unfortunately, while the first coil was placed, it poked through the weak daughter sac, which started to bleed. The bleeding confirmed that this aneurysm was responsible for the original hemorrhage. The coiling process was continued until it was established that the bleeding had stopped, which occurred within 1 to 2 minutes. The second coil further sealed the aneurysm, but obliteration was not optimal.

After 30 minutes of attempting to place coils in this aneurysm, the bleeding was well controlled. However, 3 mm of the neck of the aneurysm remained open. Repeated attempts to coil this part of the aneurysm resulted in coils bulging into the parent vessel. The bulging increased the risk of creating catastrophic blockage of that vessel. Therefore, the procedure was aborted in the patient's best interests. The microneurosurgeon recommended no further attempts at coiling the aneurysm. Placing more coils would likely eliminate the potentially clippable neck that was currently present. At this point open surgery was recommended.

By this time, N.S.'s husband had arrived in the hospital. He was made aware of her life-threatening situation, her treatment to that point, and further recommendations related to surgery. He provided informed consent on his wife's behalf to proceed with aneurysm surgery. The neurosurgeons informed her husband of both the benefits and the risks of the procedure. The risks of this procedure had increased because the team was now dealing with a ruptured aneurysm that had freshly rebled. It also had coils in it, a situation that makes it more difficult to place a clip. Nonetheless, surgery seemed the best option for N.S., because further rebleeding would likely prove fatal.

The aneurysm's neck was clipped uneventfully through a standard frontotemporal craniotomy. At the end of the procedure, the neurosurgeon reported to N.S.'s husband that her brain appeared more relaxed and that no unexpected adverse events had occurred during the operation. The coils were inside during the operation. In fact, one coil poked through the ruptured daughter sac, but it did not interfere with placing the aneurysm clip. Once the clip was placed, the endovascular surgeon repeated cerebral angiography. The scan showed that both aneurysms were obliterated. This situation gave N.S. her best chance of recovery, although she was still in critical condition.

N.S. was taken to the ICU intubated and sedated. She was weaned from sedation by the nursing staff on the first night after surgery. She was found to be able to move her right side strongly to stimulation, but her left side was weak. She was not following commands. Her postoperative CT scan showed that the right side of her brain was still swollen. However, her ICP was in the normal range. The external ventricular drain continued to drain blood-stained CSF, which relieved her ICP and ventricular system.

Over the next 7 to 8 days, N.S.'s neurological responses became stronger. She was monitored periodically for the development of cerebral vasospasm with a transcranial Doppler scalp probe. She was cared for intensively by the nursing and medical staff. Ten days after her initial hemorrhage, she began to follow commands with both sides, although her left side was still weak. A tracheostomy and a feeding tube had been placed. Even while she was semicomatose, the physical therapists and respiratory therapists had worked with her to ensure that she maintained good lung clearance via chest percussion therapy and good range of motion in her arms and legs. Her CT scans showed that most of the blood in her brain cisterns had cleared with help of the external ventricular drain. After appropriate weaning, the drain was safely discontinued. She was fortunate to have escaped the development of cerebral vasospasm and hydrocephalus.

Eventually, N.S. was transferred to the neurosurgical floor. She had become more awake by postbleed Day 13 and passed a swallow evaluation. Her feeding tube was removed. She had become strong enough to sit out of bed. Her left side was still weak but continued to improve with the help of her physical and occupational therapists.

N.S.'s scalp sutures were removed. When she was sufficiently awake and cooperative, she was transferred to the rehabilitation unit of the hospital, where she stayed another 10 days before being discharged home.

At N.S.'s 3-month postoperative visit, she had regained most of her strength. She was walking again but was not fully independent. Formal cognitive testing showed subtle impairment. She reported that her lethargy had improved considerably, but she still had some numbness over her skin incision. Her doctor informed her that she would need a few more months to maximize her overall recovery. They encouraged her to walk and to try to resume her normal daily routine.

With the aid of a supportive husband and parents, a personal mindset focused on healing and full recovery, and the close supervision of her physicians and therapists, N.S. was fortunate to have returned to her normal life within 6 months of her hemorrhage.

K.M.

At the age of 27, K.M. was brought to the emergency room by her family with complaints of increasing limb weakness, incoordination, and unsteadiness. On careful questioning she also reported some difficulty with breathing and some impairment of the strength of her voice. She added that in the past few years she had intermittently awakened with a headache and had experienced episodes of a spinning sensation or vertigo. She ascribed these episodes to her busy work life because they were infrequent. She had vomited spontaneously three times in the preceding month but had attributed it to travel or a viral illness. She had no family history of any neurological problems except for vertigo.

The neurologist examining K.M. in the emergency room found that she had mild to moderate weakness in all four limbs and unsteadiness when attempting to walk heel-to-toe like on a tight rope. He thought that her symptoms suggested that something was affecting her brainstem, such as a tumor, and ordered a brain CT scan. The CT scan showed an abnormality in the brainstem, but it was difficult to identify. An MRI, which has much higher resolution than the CT, was obtained that night. The MRI showed a round, 3-cm mass compressing and flattening the brainstem and confirmed the presence of a giant brain aneurysm. The aneurysm had probably been there for years, growing slowly, and causing the patient's recurrent and eventually progressive neurological symptoms.

The aneurysm had probably never leaked blood because K.M. had never experienced the sudden and severe headaches described by most patients with ruptured or leaking aneurysms. She was one of the few patients whose aneurysm was diagnosed from mass effect. In her case, this meant brainstem compression and mild hydrocephalus rather than rupture.

K.M. was admitted to the neurological ICU, and the next morning a cerebral angiogram was obtained. The test confirmed that the abnormality was a formidable giant aneurysm located at the vertebrobasilar junction. An endovascular surgeon and microneurosurgeon were both consulted. After careful consideration of the angiogram and of the risks associated with treating this lesion either endovascularly or by open surgery, they recommended an attempt at endovascular surgery. If that failed, K.M. would need to undergo surgery under profound hypothermia and circulatory arrest. This procedure was considered necessary during surgical exploration and treatment because of the size and location of the aneurysm and its compression of the brainstem.

While K.M. was mildly sedated for the endovascular procedure, a catheter was inserted into her right femoral artery. The catheter was advanced through the arterial system through her heart and into the arteries of her posterior circulation. Small coils and a balloon were inserted into the aneurysm and its parent artery. The balloon allowed the parent artery to be sacrificed, while the coils were placed in the dome of the aneurysm to allow it to form a clot. Based on her cerebral angiogram, K.M. had good collateral or alternate blood flow pathways to other parts of her posterior circulation. Consequently, she might be able to tolerate sacrifice of the parent artery. She was kept on a blood thinner to prevent the aneurysm from suddenly forming a clot and blocking her main brainstem artery, the basilar artery. Such a clot could have been fatal.

K.M. tolerated the procedure well and was taken to the recovery area. However, within 15 minutes, her blood pressure dropped and she experienced vertigo and speech difficulty. After treatment with more intravenous fluids, her blood pressure returned to a normal range and her symptoms improved. A repeat cerebral angiogram showed no new problem. The balloon and coils had not migrated, and the critical basilar artery was still open. She was then taken to the neurological ICU.

Over the next 3 to 4 days, K.M.'s condition worsened. The blood thinner had been weaned gradually to allow the aneurysm to clot, which CT scans confirmed. But, as the soft pulsating blood was converted to a hard, clotted mass, mass effect further compressed her brainstem. She became weaker, her heart rate began to slow, and the strength of her voice dwindled. Her physicians hoped that if she could survive this phase, the clotting process within her aneurysm would eventually cause the lesion to shrink.

Unfortunately, this process did not happen. A small amount of blood continued to flow into the aneurysm. On the seventh day after her endovascular procedure, while her husband was sitting beside her in her hospital room, K.M.'s aneurysm ruptured. Her husband recounted that she sat up in bed, stated she could not breathe, held her head in her hands, and then lay back down continuing to hold her head. The nursing staff alerted the neurosurgeon who was still in the hospital late that evening. She was taken to the CT scanner, and the scan showed that her aneurysm had leaked. Fortunately, it was not a devastating rupture.

The next morning a team of two microneurosurgeons, two cardiac surgeons, and a cardiac and neuroanesthesiologist accompanied K.M. to the operating room, where she was operated under conditions of profound hypothermia and circulatory arrest. The operation took several hours. The neurosurgeon reported that the most striking findings were that the aneurysm had shown evidence of a silent rupture. Dense clot protruded from the paper thin wall of the aneurysm in some regions. The aneurysm continued to leak intraoperatively until the moment K.M.'s heart was stopped. Stopping her heart allowed the aneurysm to be explored more safely and trapped by the neurosurgeon. No neck that could be safely clipped was present. Instead surgical clips were placed on the artery feeding the aneurysm and on the two arteries exiting the aneurysm. The aneurysm was thereby isolated from her circulation. It was then removed along with the craggy thrombus it contained. Treating a vertebrobasilar junction aneurysm in this way was associated with a high risk of brainstem stroke and death, but so did doing nothing. When her heart was restarted at the end of the procedure, her brain swelled slightly, but the swelling was rapidly controlled. The surgeons believed that the surgery had gone as well as possible but they were not sure what her condition would be when she awake.

K.M. did not awake for another 24 hours. She was kept sedated. Only intermittently was her sedation weaned briefly to see if she would move to stimulation. Fortunately, she did. Her repeat CT scan showed no new stroke and confirmed that her aneurysm was gone. Her brainstem looked more relaxed. It was no longer compressed by the aneurysm and its thrombus. K.M. was kept intubated for another 48 hours. She was now awake and following commands. All her limbs seemed strong. She was extubated 3 days after surgery. After extubation, she found it difficult to manage her own throat and airway secretions. This problem was most likely because the lower cranial nerves of the brainstem were weak from the stress of the aneurysm and its treatment. She could speak but required aggressive airway suctioning. A swallowing study showed that she had some degree of aspiration, and a nasogastric feeding tube was placed to provide her with nutrition.

During the next 4 weeks, K.M.'s condition continued to improve. She was under the care of the Physical Medicine and Rehabilitation Service. She was walking independently, her balance was improving, and her speech and swallowing had improved. Her feeding tube was removed 6 weeks after it was placed. Her strong, cheerful, and positive mindset; the care of her physicians and paramedical staff; and the close and unreserved support of her family helped her through her recovery.

K.M.'s 3-month follow-up examination showed that she had almost regained her healthy and independent baseline. A year later she delivered her first child. During her pregnancy she had already returned to her professional career. Her 5-year follow-up cerebral angiogram showed no aneurysm.

A.F.

A.F. was a healthy 48-year-old man who smoked. He experienced a sudden and severe postcoital headache that was associated with nausea and vomiting. He was taken by ambulance to the emergency room of a local teaching hospital. The evaluating physician found A.F. to be unimpaired neurologically. A head CT scan without contrast showed diffuse SAH and suggested the presence of an aneurysm at the top of the basilar artery. The neurosurgeon who evaluated A.F. in the emergency room informed him and his wife that a cerebral angiogram was needed. He explained the surgical and endovascular options for basilar apex aneurysms, and the benefits and risks of each approach. He suggested that if the aneurysm was amenable to coiling, the endovascular surgeon who performed the cerebral angiogram could coil the aneurysm at the same time. A.F. and his wife agreed with this approach. The neurosurgeon placed an external ventricular drain in A.F. before taking him to the angiography suite.

The cerebral angiogram was performed with A.F. under mild sedation rather than under general anesthesia because he was cooperative enough to hold his head still during the procedure. The angiogram showed a 7-mm aneurysm at the basilar apex. No other vascular abnormality was present. Fortunately, the aneurysm had a relatively narrow neck, and the endovascular surgeon proceeded with coiling. Three platinum microcoils were required to obliterate the aneurysm fully. Neither the parent nor surrounding arteries were compromised. The neurosurgeon informed A.F.'s wife that the procedure had gone uneventfully and that the aneurysm appeared to be treated completely. However, another angiogram would be needed in 1 year to follow the aneurysm for growth or recurrence.

A.F. was transferred to the neurological ICU where he stayed for 6 more days. Fortunately, he did not develop cerebral vasospasm, and the external ventricular drain was removed immediately before his transfer to the neurosurgical general care ward. The patient remained neurologically intact and was discharged from hospital 10 days after his admission. A follow-up appointment and angiogram with the endovascular surgeon was scheduled for 1 year later. Because of the association between smoking and brain aneurysms, A.F. was strongly advised to stop smoking.

S.C.

S.C. was a 46-year-old woman who suddenly experienced a severe headache and collapsed in her home. She was taken unconscious to the local emergency room where a head CT scan showed a massive SAH. She rapidly progressed to respiratory failure before any surgical treatment could be performed. She died, without regaining consciousness, within hours of her admission to the hospital.

CHAPTER 23.

The brain-attack and brain aneurysm alert checklist

It is widely understood that a heart attack or myocardial infarction irreversibly damages the muscle tissue of the heart through loss of its blood supply. That is, its supply of oxygen and other nutrients is severely impeded or lost as part of severe ischemia. Typically, this loss is caused by a severe fatty blockage in one or more main arteries feeding a region of the heart. The blockage can impair the heart's ability to pump blood, which can be fatal.

A brain attack is the brain's version of a heart attack. It occurs when the blood supply to a region of the brain is lost. This condition is also referred to as a stroke or cerebral infarction. Symptoms of a brain attack may be short lived. For example, a TIA may last less than 24 hours. Or the symptoms may be part of a full and permanent event, referred to as a completed stroke. The onset is typically sudden. Symptoms may include visual impairment. One symptom, called amaurosis fugax, feels like a darkish curtain has fallen across the eye. Partial or complete blindness can involve one or both eyes. There may be impairment of clarity of speech, referred to as dysarthria, or language dysfunction, referred to as dysphasia or aphasia. Impairment of limb muscle strength, known as paresis or paralysis, or impaired sensation can occur. Other symptoms include vertigo, gait imbalance, loss of consciousness, incoordination, and double vision, depending on the region of brain involved.

As in the case of the heart, the most frequent cause of loss of blood supply to brain tissue is atherosclerosis. The blood supply can also be impaired by dissection or occlusion of the carotid arteries. However, blood supply can be lost because of another important reason: a ruptured blood vessel. Consider an aneurysm. When a brain aneurysm ruptures or reruptures, the blood flowing in the parent artery from which the aneurysm arose is suddenly no longer flowing to the nerves and other cells in the brain. The blood gushes out of the vessel and into the subarachnoid space. The region of brain once supplied by the artery with the aneurysm that burst becomes ischemic. Thereafter, it may become infarcted. That is, the tissue can die. Cerebral vasospasm after aneurysmal SAH is another way in which an aneurysm may cause blood loss and hence a stroke. In this case, the stroke would be delayed.

A heart attack has a "signature," that is, the severe and prolonged crushing chest pain associated with profuse sweating, shortness of breath, and other familiar symptoms. A brain attack caused by an aneurysm also has a signature. **Table 3** is a checklist of symptoms and signs that can alert a person to the presence of an aneurysm or a hemorrhage from an aneurysm that can cause a brain attack. The list does not include every symptom or sign known to be associated with aneurysms. Rather, it includes the most common symptoms and signs. Some of these symptoms can occur in conditions unrelated to aneurysmal disease. For example, some of the symptoms can be associated with migraine, epilepsy, brain tumor, meningitis, and symptomatic carotid disease, or brain artery occlusive or inflammatory diseases.

Specific concerns should be discussed with a physician. *Time is brain.* In the event of such an emergency in the United States, one should seek medical help immediately by dialing 911.

Table 3. Unruptured and Ruptured Aneurysm Symptoms

Unruptured

New or unusual headaches (including regular morning headaches)

Unexplained nausea and vomiting

Headache with neck stiffness

Neurological impairment (e.g., new double vision, episodic loss of vision, vertigo [dizziness], limb weakness, gait imbalance)

New onset seizure disorder

Ruptured

Sudden, excruciating headache (including during emotional or physical strain, sexual activity)

Headache with neck stiffness

Sudden neurological impairment (including one-sided body weakness or physical collapse)

CHAPTER 24.
References and resources

Literature references

Several references have been chosen as recommended reading for each topic. Many other excellent books and articles could have been included. The ones listed below were selected as a suitable introduction to, or overview of, a specific topic.

Structure and function of brain arteries

- Primer on Cerebrovascular Diseases (Textbook). Edited by Welch KMA, Caplan LR, Reis DJ, Siesjo BK, Weir B. Published by Academic Press (San Diego, CA). 1997.

- VG Khurana, JA Friedman, FB Meyer: Chapter 11: Biology of Cerebral Blood Vessels and Blood Flow. In Le Roux PD, Winn HR, Newell DW (eds), Management of Cerebral Aneurysms (Textbook), Philadelphia, WB Saunders, pp 139-167, 2004.

- RM Lee. Morphology of cerebral arteries. *Pharmacology and Therapeutics*. Volume **6 Suppl 4**. Pages 149-173. 1995.

- E Dahl. The ultrastructure of cerebral blood vessels in man. *Cephalalgia*. Volume **6**. Pages 45-48. 1986.

- JE Brian Jr, FM Faraci, DD Heistad. Recent insights into the regulation of the cerebral circulation. *Clinical and Experimental Pharmacology and Physiology.* Volume **23**. Pages 449-457. 1996.

- M Wahl, L Schilling. Regulation of cerebral blood flow - A brief review. *Acta Neurochirurgica Suppl (Wien).* Volume **59**. Pages 3-10. 1993.

Brain aneurysms

- Pathology of the Cerebral Blood Vessels (Textbook). Written by Stehbens WE. Published by CV Mosby (St. Louis, MO). 1972.

- J Suzuki, H Ohara. Clinicopathological study of cerebral aneurysms: Origin, rupture, repair, and growth. *Journal of Neurosurgery.* Volume **48**. Pages 505-514. 1978.

- Aneurysms Affecting the Nervous System (Textbook). Written by Weir B. Published by Williams & Wilkins (Baltimore, MD). 1987.

- Giant Intracranial Aneurysms (Textbook). Edited by Awad IA, Barrow D. Published by the American Association of Neurological Surgeons (AANS) Publications Committee (Park Ridge, IL). 1995.

- MT Lawton, RF Spetzler. Surgical strategies for giant intracranial aneurysms. *Neurosurgery Clinics of North America.* Volume **9**. Pages 725-742. 1998.

- SP Javedan SP, VR Deshmukh, RF Spetzler, JM Zabramski. The role of cerebral revascularization in patients with intracranial aneurysms. *Neurosurgery Clinics of North America.* Volume **12**. Pages 541-555. 2001.

- JJ Evans, LN Sekhar, R Rak, D Stimac. Bypass grafting and revascularization in the management of posterior circulation aneurysms. *Neurosurgery.* Volume **55**. Pages 1036-1049. 2004.

- DG Peters, AB Kassam, E Feingold, E Heidrich-O'Hare, H Yonas, RE Ferrell, A Brufsky. Molecular anatomy of an intracranial aneurysm: Coordinated expression of genes involved in wound healing and tissue remodeling. *Stroke.* Volume **32**. Pages 1036-1042, 2001.

- VG Khurana, I Meissner, FB Meyer. Update on genetic evidence for rupture-prone compared with rupture-resistant intracranial saccular aneurysms. *Neurosurgical Focus.* Volume **17**. E7. 2004.

- WI Schievink. Intracranial aneurysms. *New England Journal of Medicine.* Volume **336**. Pages 28-40. 1997.

- GJ Rinkel, M Djibuti, A Algra, J van Gijn. Prevalence and risk of rupture of intracranial aneurysms: A systematic review. *Stroke.* Volume **29**. Pages 251-256. 1998.

Unruptured brain aneurysms

- International Study of Unruptured Intracranial Aneurysms (ISUIA) Investigators. Unruptured intracranial aneurysms: Risks of rupture and risks of surgical intervention. *New England Journal of Medicine.* Volume **339**. Pages 1725-1733. 1998.

- DO Wiebers, JP Whisnant, WM O'Fallon. The natural history of unruptured intracranial aneurysms. *New England Journal of Medicine.* Volume **304**. Pages 696-698. 1981.

- DO Wiebers, JP Whisnant, TM Sundt Jr, et al. The significance of unruptured intracranial saccular aneurysms. *Journal of Neurosurgery.* Volume **66**. Pages 23-29. 1987.

- LR Caplan. Should intracranial aneurysms be treated before they rupture? *New England Journal of Medicine.* Volume **339**. Pages 1774-1775. 1998.

- JB Bederson, IA Awad, DO Wiebers, et al. Recommendations for the management of patients with unruptured intracranial aneurysms: A statement for healthcare professionals from the Stroke Council of the American Heart Association. *Circulation*. Volume **102**. Pages 2300-2308. 2000.

- VG Khurana, I Meissner, YR Sohni, WR Bamlet, RL McClelland, JM Cunningham, FB Meyer. The presence of tandem endothelial nitric oxide synthase gene polymorphisms identifying brain aneurysms more prone to rupture. *Journal of Neurosurgery*. Volume **102**. Pages 526-531. 2005.

Aneurysmal bleeding and rebleeding

- TM Sundt Jr, JP Whisnant. Subarachnoid hemorrhage from intracranial aneurysms. Surgical management and natural history of disease. *New England Journal of Medicine*. Volume **299**. Pages 116-122. 1978.

- NF Kassell, JC Torner. Aneurysmal rebleeding: A preliminary report from the Cooperative Aneurysm Study. *Neurosurgery*. Volume **13**. Pages 479-481. 1983.

- VG Khurana, DG Piepgras, JP Whisnant JP. Ruptured giant intracranial aneurysms. Part I. A study of rebleeding. *Journal of Neurosurgery*. Volume **88**. Pages 425-429. 1998.

- DG Piepgras, VG Khurana, DA Nichols. Occult rupture of a giant vertebral artery aneurysm following proximal occlusion and intrasaccular thrombosis. Case report. *Journal of Neurosurgery*. Volume **95**. Pages 132-137. 2001.

- J Hillman, C von Essen, W Leszniewski, I Johansson. Significance of "ultra-early" rebleeding in subarachnoid hemorrhage. *Journal of Neurosurgery*. Volume **68**. Pages 901-907. 1988.

- RD Verweij, EFM Wijdicks, J van Gijn. Warning headache in aneurysmal subarachnoid hemorrhage. A case-control study. *Archives of Neurology*. Volume **45**. Pages 1019-1020. 1988.

A study of clipping versus coiling ruptured aneurysms, and the critique of International Subarachnoid Aneurysm Trial

- AJ Molyneux, RS Kerr, LM Yu, M Clarke, M Sneade, JA Yarnold, P Sandercock, et al. International subarachnoid aneurysm trial (ISAT) of neurosurgical clipping versus endovascular coiling in 2143 patients with ruptured intracranial aneurysms: A randomized comparison of effects on survival, dependency, seizures, rebleeding, subgroups, and aneurysmal occlusion. *Lancet*. Volume **366**. Pages 809-817. 2005.

- GW Britz. ISAT trial: Coiling or clipping for intracranial aneurysms? *Lancet*. Volume **366**. Pages 783-785. 2005.

Cerebral vasospasm

- B Weir. The pathophysiology of cerebral vasospasm. *British Journal of Neurosurgery*. Volume **9**. Pages 375-390. 1995.

- HH Dietrich, RG Dacey Jr. Molecular keys to the problems of cerebral vasospasm. *Neurosurgery*. Volume **46**. Pages 517-530. 2000.

- B Weir, L MacDonald. Cerebral vasospasm. *Clinical Neurosurgery*. Volume **40**. Pages 40-55. 1993.

- NWC Dorsch, MT King. A review of cerebral vasospasm in aneurysmal subarachnoid haemorrhage. Part I. Incidence and effects. *Journal of Clinical Neuroscience*. Volume **1**. Pages 19-26. 1994.

- VG Khurana, M Besser. Pathophysiological basis of cerebral vasospasm following aneurysmal subarachnoid haemorrhage. *Journal of Clinical Neuroscience*. Volume **4**. Pages 122-131. 1997.

- VG Khurana, YR Sohni, WI Mangrum, RL McClelland, DJ O'Kane, FB Meyer, I Meissner. Endothelial nitric oxide synthase gene polymorphisms predict susceptibility to aneurysmal subarachnoid hemorrhage and cerebral vasospasm. *Journal of Cerebral Blood Flow and Metabolism*. Volume **24**. Pages 291-297. 2004.

- IA Awad, LP Carter, RF Spetzler, M Medina, FC Williams Jr. Clinical vasospasm after subarachnoid hemorrhage: Response to hypervolemic hemodilution and arterial hypertension. *Stroke*. Volume **18**. Pages 365-72. 1987.

Cerebral blood flow and metabolism

- Cerebral Blood Flow and Metabolism (Textbook). Written by L Edvinsson, ET Mackenzie, J McCulloch. Published by Raven Press (New York, NY). 1993.

- VG Khurana, EE Benarroch, ZS Katusic, FB Meyer: Chapter 86: Cerebral Blood Flow and Metabolism. In Winn HR (ed), Youmans Neurological Surgery, 5th Edition, Vol. 2, Philadelphia, WB Saunders, pp 1467-1494, 2003.

- Brain Energy Metabolism (Textbook). Written by BK Siesjo. Published by John Wiley & Sons (New York, NY). 1978.

- Neurosurgery Clinics of North America: Cerebral Blood Flow (Serial-Text). Volume 7. Edited by FB Meyer. Published by WB Saunders (Philadelphia, PA). 1996.

- FM Faraci, JE Brian. Nitric oxide and the cerebral circulation. *Stroke*. Volume **25**. Pages 692-703. 1994.

- SS Kety. The circulation, metabolism, and functional activity of the human brain. *Neurochemical Research*. Volume **16**. Pages 1073-1078. 1991.

Nitric Oxide and eNOS

- S Moncada, RMJ Palmer, EA Higgs. Nitric oxide: Physiology, pathophysiology, and pharmacology. *Pharmacological Reviews*. Volume **43**. Pages 109-142. 1991.

- S Moncada, A Higgs. The L-arginine-nitric oxide pathway. *New England Journal of Medicine*. Volume **329**. Pages 2002-2012. 1993.

- E Anggard. Nitric oxide: Mediator, murderer, and medicine. *Lancet*. Volume **343**: 1199-1206. 1994.

- PA Marsden, HHQ Heng, SW Scherer, RJ Stewart, AV Hall, XM Shi, LC Tsui, KT Schappert. Structure and chromosomal localization of the human constitutive endothelial nitric oxide synthase gene. *Journal of Biological Chemistry*. Volume **268**. Pages 17478-17488. 1993.

- T Dalkara, MA Moskowitz. Nitric oxide and the cerebral circulation. In: KMA Welch, LR Caplan, DJ Reis, BK Siesjo, B Weir (editors): Primer on Cerebrovascular Diseases. San Diego, CA. Academic Press. Pages 96-98. 1997.

- XL Wang, J Wang. Endothelial nitric oxide synthase gene sequence variations and vascular disease. *Molecular Genetics and Metabolism*. Volume **70**. Pages 241-251. 2000.

Genomics

- JM Rusnak, RM Kisabeth, DP Herbert, DM McNeil. Pharmacogenomics: A clinician's primer on emerging technologies for improved patient care. *Mayo Clinic Proceedings*. Volume **76**. Pages 299-309. 2001.

- WE Evans, MV Relling. Pharmacogenomics: Translating functional genomics into rational therapeutics. *Science*. Volume **286**. Pages 487-491. 1999.

- AD Roses. Genetic susceptibility to cardiovascular diseases. *American Heart Journal*. Volume **140**. Pages S45-S47. 2000.

- EM Rubin, A Tall. Perspectives for vascular genomics. *Nature*. Volume **407**. Pages 265-269. 2000.

- CP Lorentz, ED Wieben, A Tefferi, DA Whiteman, GW Dewald. Primer on medical genomics. Part I: History of genetics and sequencing of the human genome. *Mayo Clinic Proceedings*. Volume **77**. Pages 773-782. 2002.

- A Pardanani, ED Wieben, TC Spelsberg, A Tefferi. Primer on medical genomics. Part IV: Expression proteomics. *Mayo Clinic Proceedings*. Volume **77**. Pages 1185-1196. 2002.

- SM Ansell, MJ Ackerman, JL Black, LR Roberts, A Tefferi. Primer on medical genomics. Part VI: Genomics and molecular genetics in clinical practice. *Mayo Clinic Proceedings*. Volume **78**. Pages 307-317. 2003.

Gene therapy and cerebrovascular gene transfer

- HM Blau, ML Springer. Gene therapy - A novel form of drug delivery. *New England Journal of Medicine*. Volume **333**. Pages 1204-1207. 1995.

- MA Kay, JC Glorioso, L Naldini. Viral vectors for gene therapy: The art of turning infectious agents into vehicles of therapeutics. *Nature Medicine*. Volume 7. Pages 33-40. 2001.

- MR Dyer, PL Herrling. Progress and potential for gene-based medicines. *Molecular Therapy*. Volume **1**. Pages 213-224. 2000.

- DD Heistad, FM Faraci. Gene therapy for cerebral vascular disease. *Stroke*. Volume **27**. Pages 1688-1693. 1996.

- AFY Chen, T O'Brien, ZS Katusic. Transfer and expression of recombinant nitric oxide synthase genes in the cardiovascular system. *Trends in Pharmacological Sciences*. Volume **19**. Pages 276-286. 1998.

- VG Khurana, FB Meyer. Translational paradigms in cerebrovascular gene transfer. *Journal of Cerebral Blood Flow and Metabolism*. Volume **23**. Pages 1251-1262. 2003.

- VG Khurana, LA Smith, TA Baker, D Eguchi, T O'Brien, ZS Katusic. Protective vasomotor effects of in vivo recombinant endothelial nitric oxide synthase gene expression in a canine model of cerebral vasospasm. *Stroke*. Volume **33**. Pages 782-789. 2002.

Internet resources

The following URLs may provide useful information for patients with brain aneurysms and other disorders.

- **Brain-aneurysm.com**. A comprehensive Site on brain blood vessels and their disorders. http://www.brain-aneurysm.com

- **The Barrow Neurological Institute** (BNI). The BNI Website has information on numerous medical disorders, including brain aneurysm, and specialist services. http://www.thebni.com

- **The Mayo Clinic**. The Mayo Website also has helpful information on numerous medical disorders and specialist services. http://www.mayoclinic.com

- **Brain Aneurysm Foundation**. A resourceful organization providing an aneurysm support network. http://bafound.org/

- **Aneurysm & AVM Support**. A Site with helpful aneurysm and AVM resources and links, including many patient stories. http://www.westga.edu/%7ewmaples/

- **Brain Storm**. A collection of resources, including many links, related to brain aneurysms. http://www2.canisius.edu/%7eemeryg/brain.html

- **Neurosurgery On-Call**. The premier U.S. neurosurgical professional and public Site on the Web. http://www.neurosurgery.org/

- **Cerebrovascular Surgery Division**. Home of the AANS & CNS division concerned with cerebrovascular surgery. http://www.neurosurgery.org/cv

- **American Association of Neurological Surgeons** (AANS). Home of one of the two main neurosurgical professional societies in the United States. http://www.aans.org/

- **Congress of Neurological Surgeons** (CNS). Home of one of the two main neurosurgical professional societies in the United States. http://www.neurosurgeon.org/

- **World Federation of Neurosurgical Societies** (WFNS). Home of the main world-wide neurosurgical professional society. http://wfns.org/

- **American Heart Association** (AHA). The premier U.S. cardiovascular disease professional and public Site on the Web. http://www.americanheart.org/

- **AHA - American Stroke Association** (ASA). Home of the division of the AHA concerned with diseases of the brain circulation. http://www.strokeassociation.org/

- **PubMed Literature Search**. Search engine of the National Institutes of Health (NIH) for medical journal articles. http://www.pubmed.com